Clinical guidelines

Diagnostic
and treatment manual

for curative programs
in rural hospitals, dispensaries
and refugee camps

for the use of doctors and nurses

1993 – THIRD EDITION

Clinical guidelines

Diagnostic and treatment manual

EDITOR :

J.C. DESENCLOS (MD)

THIRD EDITION COORDINATED BY

P. BIBERSON (MD)
J. RIGAL (MD)

Contributions (in alphabetical order) :

H. Audrain (N), P. Autier (MD), M.J. de Chazelles (Oph), J. Combreau (MW),
E. Couturier (MD), B. Faucher (MD), V. Fauveau (MD), L. Flachet (MD),
A. Fourrier (Ph), J.J. Frère (MD), D. Jorland (CD), J. Lagoutte (MD),
A. Moren (MD), B. Morinière (MD), F. Mounis (O), B. Pécoul (MD), J. Pinel (Ph),
M. Postel (MD), B. Renchon (Ph), V. Schwœbel (MD), C. Ségala (MD),
P. Sotias (MD), V. Van Stirtegheim (MD).

FRENCH-ENGLISH TRANSLATION COORDINATED BY

P. HAKEWILL (MD)
J. PORTER (MD)
R. KESSEL (MD)

*(MD) Medical doctor, (MW) Midwife, (N) Nurse, (O) Osteopath, (Ph) Pharmacist, (D) Dentist,
(Opht) Ophthalmologist*

We would like to thank Dr S. Sorensen (Essential drugs program, WHO),
Professor M. Rey (WHO and Dr Houlemarre (Centre International de
l'Enfance) for their advice and suggestions ; Dr G. Desvé, Mr M. Pottier
and Miss O. Hardy for their technical assistance in the writing or this
manual.

This book would not have been possible without Ms Evelyne LAISSU who
was responsible for the design and layout.

Foreword

This clinical manual is a collective work, for daily field practice.

We have tried to incorporate information from various sources : the field experience of Médecins sans Frontières personnel, the recommendations from reference institutions such as World Health Organization (W.H.O.) and from text books and monographs most relevant to the domain of medical care in developing countries (see bibliography, page 313).

This manual is for doctors, nurses and other health professionals responsible for curative care in rural dispensaries and hospitals, as well as in displace people or refugee camps.

It covers the curative and to a lesser extent the preventive aspects of the main conditions encountered in the field. It should function as a supportive tool towards the elaboration of an adapted health policy. The introduction of this manual will emphasize the basis of such a policy.

With a view to future revisions and to keep the work as close as possible to field realities, the authors would be grateful for critical comments and suggestions from users of this manual.

Comments should be send to

Médecins sans Frontières – Service médical
8 rue Saint-Sabin – 75544 Paris Cedex 11 – France
Tel. : (33.1) 40.21.29.29 – Fax : (33.1) 48.06.68.68 – Tlx : 214 360 F

How to use these guidelines

Organisation

The information you are looking for can be found :

1. At the beginning of the manual in the table of *contents* : numbers of chapters with page numbers.
2. At the end of the manual in the *alphabetical index* whith the lists all diseases

Abbreviations used

mg	=	milligramme		PO	=	per os (orally)
g	=	gramme		IM	=	intramuscular
kg	=	kilogramme		IV	=	intravenous
d	=	day		SC	=	subcutaneous
x	=	times		IU	=	international units
stat	=	at once ; one single dose		MIU	=	million international units

AFB	=	acid fast bacilli		PR	=	per rectum
BP	=	blood pressure		PV	=	per vaginam
CCF	=	congestive cardiac failure		PUO	=	pyrexia of unknown origin
CSF	=	cerebrospinal fluid		RBC	=	red blood cell
GIT	=	gastro-intestinal tract		RR	=	respiratory rate
Hct	=	hæmatocrit		RTI	=	respiratory tract infection
MCH	=	maternal-child health		spp	=	species
ORS	=	oral rehydration salts		STD	=	sexually transmitted diseases
ORT	=	oral rehydration therapy		TB	=	Tuberculosis
PID	=	pelvic inflammatory disease		WBC	=	white blood cell

– Cotrimoxazole = mixture of sulfamethoxazole (SMX) + Trimetoprim (TMP)
  Usual dosage is : 400 mg SMX + 80 mg TMP

– Peni G = Benzyl penicillin = Crystalline penicillin G

– PPF = Fortified procaine penicillin = mixture of procain benzyl penicillin and Benzyl penicillin

Conversion °C into °F : remove 2, multiply by 2, add 30
Conversion °F into °C : remove 30, divide by 2, add 2

International non proprietary name for drugs

The International Non-proprietary Name (INN) of drugs is used in this manual. A list of equivalent commercial running name can be found page 311.

Contents

INTRODUCTION

In a health program adapted to the needs of a developing country, the curative care is an important component. Initially however, more important measures have to be implemented to provide the foundations for all programs aimed at improving the health of a community. These measures are related to :
– sanitation,
– nutrition,
– hygiene,
– immunization,
– maternal and child health,
– health education,
– health workers training,
– community awareness and participation.

These measures should interact and complement the curative care component of the health program.

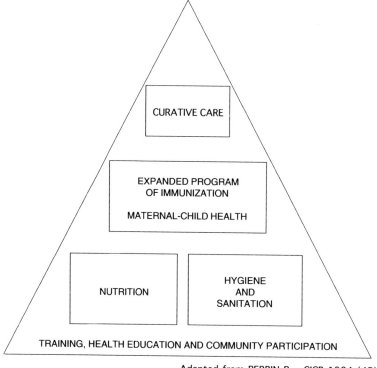

Adapted from PERRIN P. - CICR 1984 (45)

Figure 1
Structure of a health service

Objectives for a curative health program

At the individual level

The objective is to cure the patient and to minimize or prevent the consequences of illness (eg. transmission).

At the community level

The objectives are to reduce the mortality and morbidity attributable to the common severe illnesses in the community.

For a few infectious endemic diseases

Curative care can reduce transmission of certain diseases (e.g. TB, leprosy, trypanosomiasis, bilharzia) provided a high proportion of the infected community is treated.

Strategy

In developing countries there are enormous needs and limited resources. The resources should be aimed at the diseases, amenable to effective treatment in the field, which are causing high mortality and morbidity (priority diseases).

Priority diseases can vary from one geographical region to another, but a standard epidemiological profile remains. In order to get an accurate profile an initial assessment is necessary. It should be qualitative (descriptive), and if possible, quantitative (incidence, morbidity and mortality rates). This evaluation will characterise the most common diseases (e.g. diarrhoea, acute respiratory infections...) and will identify the exposed and high risk groups in the population (e.g. children < 5 years, pregnant women...). These diseases and high risk groups should be the targets of the program. This does not mean that curative care should be limited to these diseases and groups of people, but rather that the resources, particularly at the primary health care level, should be targeted at these groups.

In some instances (e.g. displaced or isolated persons) a complete evaluation is necessary. In other instances, such as a rehabilitation program or a study to reinforce an existing program, the Ministry of Health (MOH) may already have qualitative or quantitative data available and only a partial evaluation may be necessary.

The health care program can be defined and carried out as soon as priorities have been defined, and health policy and local resources identified (e.g. essential drug list, MOH management protocols, medical personnel and their training and the medical structure).
This manual, *"Essential drugs - practical guidelines"* (22) and *"Principales conduites à tenir en dispensaire"* (23) are additional tools to help evaluate, define and establish a health care program (e.g. management protocols, training, guidelines...).

Health care organization

In certain situations (e.g. displaced populations, refugees), a program has to be created, whereas in others, an existing program is evaluated so it can be improved.

Infrastructure and medical staff

Health centers, dispensaries, medical centers and hospitals are run by personnel with different skills and different levels of competence (e.g. community health workers (C.H.W.), medical auxiliaries, nurses, midwifes and doctors).
The evaluation should clarify their technical level. In refugee camps, most of the staff will have no previous training.

Medicines

Selection of medicines depends on the targets and needs identified in the epidemiological profile. However, are other restraints : cost, stability, administration route, duration of treatment and whether single or multiple drug doses are required.
The W.H.O. list of essential drugs (appendix 3, page 265), is the basic framework for establishing an essential drug list. A drug list should be defined in accordance with objectives, target diseases, epidemiological profile, medical staff competence and whether it is possible to refer severe cases. The quantitative and qualitative drug lists of the Emergency Health Kit (for 10.000 persons for 3 months) recommended by the W.H.O. and Médecins sans Frontières are given as an example in appendix 4 (page 271).
Drugs are listed under their International Nonproprietary (generic) Names : INN.

Therapeutic protocols

These protocols are the foundation stone of any curative health program and should be standardised in order to have an effective impact on the target diseases.
The therapeutic protocols should :
– Give clear accurate instructions.
– Include the therapeutic uses and dosages of drugs, and the duration of treatment.
– Choose the most effective drug with least side effects.
– Be supported by epidemiological and clinical data and should be discussed and agreed by the users.
– Be practical, simple, understandable and adapted to the field.
– Encourage the training and retraining of medical staff.
– Encourage the organization of medical infrastructure (e.g. pharmacy, management...).
– Be periodically re-evaluated.
– Always use the national recommendations of the country.

The therapeutic protocols should be adapted to the skill and knowledge of the medical staff. They should cover : drug prescription, curative and preventive measures, cases which should be notified (e.g. epidemic threats : cholera, typhoid), and the grounds for referral to a superior level hospital.
Protocols should be adapted to :

1) The skill and knowledge of the medical staff
   A doctor is trained in terms of diseases and syndromes (e.g. pneumonia, liver abscess) whereas a Community Health Worker (CHW) is trained in terms of symptoms (e.g. cough, fever). These two approaches are presented in Chapter 2 "Respiratory Diseases", with an introduction of the WHO program on respiratory conditions (38) which is founded on a symptomatic approach (see pages 45-49).

2) The cultural milieu and environment
   For example, if it is the custom to treat children with diarrhea with rice water, or for children with fevers to remain clothed, do not reprimand their parents.

3) The pharmaceutical supplies and local dosages of drugs
   Dosages are often different between countries (e.g. chloroquine 100 mg or 150 mg tablets).

4) The improvement of patient treatment and compliance
   It is recommended that prescribed treatments are short (< 5 days) and, if possible, in single or twice daily doses. "Stat dose" treatments, although less effective pharmacologically, do not rely on patient compliance (e.g. treat amœbiasis with a single dose of 8 metronidazole tablets (tab 250 mg) instead of a 7 day course). For the same reasons, the prescription should be limited to a maximum of 2 prescribed drugs. Injections should be avoided to reduce HIV transmission (see pages 172-180) or B hepatitis (see pages 170-171).

Protocols should avoid classical mistakes like recommending the boiling of water when energy resources (e.g. wood) are limited.

Recommendations and examples of therapeutic protocols can be found in :

- The protocols from the "New Emergency Health Kit" (CHW level) to target diseases (see appendix 4, page 271).
- The clinical and treatment sections of this manual.

Diagnostic methods

These methods depend on the structure of the organization and on the technical expertise of the staff. Staff expertise directly influences protocol formulation and drug list contents.

As a rule, diagnosis is based on the clinical examination and basic laboratory investigations (as it is defined in WHO).

Clinical examination

The principles here described are for trained medical staff. The approach for the CHW is similar but simpler.

Quality history taking and clinical examination is vital. If poor, the process from syndrome etiology to diagnosis will likewise be poor, and the treatment inappropriate. It is important to master a technique of clinical assessment that is methodical, complete and rapid. A method is all the more necessary because in field conditions the laboratory support may be rudimentary and the practitioner may have to communicate with the patient via an interpreter.

The following examination framework should be adapted to conditions. It emphasizes the advantages of a methodical approach.

CIRCUMSTANCES OF THE EXAMINATION

- *Routine*, as in a MCH clinic for prenatal women and well babies. The emphasis of the examination will depend upon local circumstances eg prevalence of anemia, malnutrition.
- *With respect to a complaint*, the commonest of which tend to be pain, fever, cough, diarrhea, fatigue...

APPROACH TO HISTORY AND PHYSICAL EXAMINATION

- A methodical approach is vital. This will save time and reduce omissions.
- An interpreter will usually be necessary. He/she must have received prior training and there must be good rapport between the clinician and the interpreter. Eventually, a good interpreter takes a very active role in the clinical process and becomes far more than a simple translator. Choosing an interpreter requires thought ; the person must be acceptable to the community and appropriate for the specific role (eg a woman for obstetrics and gynæcology).
- Learning the local words for major symptoms and diseases will allow the clinician to check that an interpreter, unfamilar to him or her (such as a relative), is giving an accurate rendition of the patient's complaints.

FRAMEWORK OF A CLINICAL ASSESSMENT

- *History*
  - history of the present illness
  - the circumstances
  - past history, family history
  - current medications, allergies
- *Examination*
  The patient should be undressed if possible.
  - General appearance : nutrition (weight and height of children), hydration, temperature, pallor ; does the patient look sick ?
  - Examination by systems : respiratory, cardiovascular, etc. This part of the examination in particular should be rigorously methodical.

- *Laboratory Tests* : if necessary.
- *Diagnosis* : This is a synthesis of all information gathered from the history, physical examination and laboratory tests. A diagnosis should be etiological but may of necessity be only symptomatic.
- *Treatment*
  - etiological, ie treating the cause. This may have to await the results of laboratory results ;
  - symptomatic ;
  - advice to the patient, whether or not a treatment is given.
- All important clinical data should be recorded, either on a card or in a family health booklet. Especially note positive and significant negative clinical signs, laboratory results, and treatment given (generic name, dose, duration).

Role of the laboratory

A basic medical laboratory of the type described by WHO can play an important role. Nevertheless, there are special constraints upon the operation of a laboratory, which should not be underestimated. There are staff constraints (necessity of trained and competent technicians), logistic constraints (supply of reagents and other equipment), time constraints (a minimum of time is necessary for each examination) and quality constraints. If attention is not paid to the above considerations, the laboratory will loose its accuracy and therefore its useful purpose.
Two levels of examination should be considered :

BASIC EXAMINATION

- Stool exams direct and stained with Lugol's iodine solution, for parasites (ova, cysts, protozoa…).
- Blood slides : thick and thin smears (for malaria, trypanosomiasis, filiariasis, relapsing fever, screening for leucocytes) : GIEMSA stain.
- Hemoglobin (Lovibond method).
- Urine exam :
  - urine analysis : dipsticks for glucose and proteins.
- Sputum exam : Ziehl - Nielsen stain.
- Urethral and vaginal swabs : slides for gonococcus and trichomonas.
- CSF exam

COMPLEX EXAMINATIONS

Certain more complex examinations may be provided according to the specific program.

A laboratory can be used in two complementary ways :

- *Clinically* : examinations can be requested for individual patients according to the clinical picture. The aim will be to assist the practitioner in :
  • diagnosis orientation (e.g. leucocytosis in blood count) ;
  • etiological diagnosis (e.g. stool exam for parasites, malaria smear...).

- *Epidemiologically* : the aim will be to construct or to validate clinical and therapeutic protocols. One can investigate a sample of patients presenting with a particular clinical picture (symptoms and syndromes) specify the etiology of that clinical picture and thus arrive at an appropriate standardized therapeutic management protocol.
  For example :
  • Fever and chills : are they due to malaria ? Rather than being obliged to perform blood slides on every febrile patient, choose at random 100 patients presenting with these symptoms and investigate them. If a significant proportion of the blood slides are positive, such cases can henceforth be presumed to be malaria and treated according to an appropriate protocol.
  • Bloody or mucusy diarrhea with no fever : the same approach can be used to determine if this clinical presentation is synonymous with amœbiasis and/or another intestinal parasite.
  • This epidemiological method of using a laboratory is especially appropriate in responding to priority needs. It can be used in emergency or "normal" conditions. Bibliographical references n° 2 and 19 give two examples for malaria, one in a refugee camp, another one in Malawi.

The training

Training or retraining of medical staff should be directed at program objectives and means (e.g. target diseases, list of essential drugs, management protocols) and should take into consideration the technical level of the staff (to be evaluated). The training program should be defined according to local needs.

Community awareness and participation

It is necessary for curative care to cover the whole population and target diseases. Coverage should be as wide as possible.

For many reasons (e.g. ignorance, different cultural perception), a large proportion of severely ill patients may present late or may pass through the system without being cured. Coverage can be improved by increasing awareness, improving health education, encouraging the exchange of information at all levels and by improving the quality of care.

Management

Consider how to efficiently and effectively manage available resources.
Figure 2 gives an example of organization of an out-patient department.

Evaluation

The evaluation of the common diseases and their effects on the community directly influence the nature of a program.

Program evaluation should be performed at the following levels :

– *Level of functioning*

Activity assessment, quantity of drugs used, prescription management, correct use of protocols, pharmacy management (orders, reports and stock keeping), all of this information should be used as indicators in program management. The morbidity rate at the dispensary level and its analysis is a useful epidemiological observation. Target disease variation in the community can be followed according to time, place, and population concerned (eg. : morbidity survey, appendix 2, page 259).

– *Level of coverage*

The aim is to determine what proportion of all patients affected by target diseases are reached by the program. Good coverage is an essential factor. The evaluation should be done on a representative sample of a target population (see below).

– *Level of community impact*

This aspect is difficult to evaluate. The evaluation relates to the objectives and should be expressed in terms of a decrease in morbidity and/or mortality. A mortality survey of a community can be conducted over a defined period of time. If the total population is known, a mortality rate can be determined.

Sample protocols for community surveys are available and have been used for evaluations (e.g. WHO, diarrheal disease program ((37)), but they require much organization and need to be repeated to give evidence of a trend).

Figure 2 : *organization of curative service*   (in order to simplify the diagram, the laboratory is not shown)

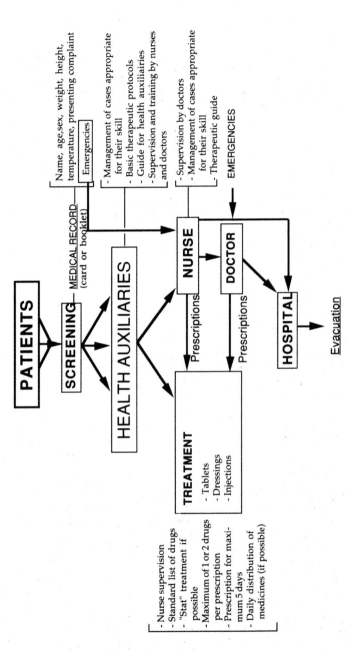

CHAPTER 1

A few symptoms and syndromes

Fatigue

☞ Fatigue is **one of the commonest** presenting complaints. The term includes various subjective symptoms (lassitude, lack of energy etc), that are both physical and mental. In most of cases there is no pathological basis to be found, however **it must not be forgotten that many diseases** may present as fatigue. The symptom, as much as any other, requires a full, **methodical** clinical assessment.

Clinical features

The history and physical examination must define :

- **Mode of onset** : sudden or progressive, old or recent, isolated or associated with other symptoms, life situation (work, intense activity, recent illness, refugee displacement...).

- **Nature of the fatigue** : physical, intellectual, sexual... ; whether it comes on in the morning (often psychosomatic) or evening (more usual).

- **Any associated clinical features** :
  • Systemic features : anorexia, weight loss, fever, anaemia, all of which suggest a probable organic basis.
  • Localizing features linked to a particular organ system, eg cough and hæmoptysis in TB, dyspnea in cardiac failure or anaemia, abdominal pains in parasitoses, jaundice in hepatitis.

- **Physical findings : the examination must be comprehensive** :
  • Nutritional status : weight (signs of recent loss), anaemia, signs of vitamin deficiency diseases...
  • Cardiopulmonary : pulse, BP, chest auscultation...
  • Abdomen : including liver, spleen...
  • Lymph nodes
  • Skin and mucus membranes
  • Affect : anxiety, depression.

Diagnosis and Treatment *(dispensary)*

- **If the fatigue is part of a syndrome**, treat the cause.

- If there seems to be **no organic basis**, assume the complaint is psychosomatic. Advise the patient to consult a traditional healer, who is usually in a far better position to help. Depending on national recommendations, a placebo may be prescribed, give :
  multivitamins : 1 tab x 3/d x 5 days.

Pain

 Pain is a common presenting symptom and of course may be caused by a range of conditions. Pain is a subjective experience. The same degree of pain will be expressed differently from patient to patient. There are also cultural differences. The assessment of the severity of pain in a given patient is thus difficult. The solution is to address the problem with a clinical approach that is both methodical and comprehensive.

Clinical features

The history of the pain elicited from the patient must define :
- Onset : sudden, subacute or progressive.
- Duration.
- Localization and radiation.
- Nature of the pain : colicky, burning, sharp, constricting, like a weight ; and whether intermittent or continuous.
- Factors that induce or relieve the pain : posture, coughing, deep breaths, meals, specific foods, movement etc.
- Associated systemic features : fever, fatigue, weight loss, etc.
- Associated focal features : cough, diarrhea, vomiting, burning during micturition...

The physical examination should be oriented towards the organ system or region where the pain seems to be localized. The synthesis of the clinical data provides the diagnosis and orients therapy, both etiological and symptomatic.

Treatment

ETIOLOGICAL

That is, treatment of the cause of the pain.

SYMPTOMATIC *(dispensary)*

According to the nature of the pain.
- *Headache*
  acetylsalicylic acid (PO) : 3 g/d divided in 3 doses x 3-5 days
  or
  paracetamol (PO) : 1.5 g/d divided in 3 doses x 3-5 days

– *Psychosomatic pains* : consider this diagnosis if pains are multiple, fleeting, or shifting. Treat as for headache or refer to a traditional healer.

– *Joint pains*
acetylsalicylic acid (PO) :
Adult : 3 g/d divided in 3 doses x 3-5 days
Child : 50 mg/kg/d divided in 3 doses x 3-5 days

– *Inflammatory* : tends to be worse at night. Look for an infectious cause (may require surgical drainage and antibiotics).
If acetylsalicylic acid is ineffective, treat with :
indomethacin (PO) :
Adult : 50 to 150 mg/d divided in 3 doses x 3-5 days

– *Joint pain (especially monoarticular)* : exclude septic arthritis. Note that periarticular and bone pains with swelling and loss of function of the limb may be due to scurvy : look for bleeding from the gums and treat with :
Ascorbic acid (vitamin C) (PO) :
Adult : 500 to 1,000 mg/d divided in 3 doses until recovery
Child : 100 to 300 mg/d divided in 3 doses until recovery
Give dietary Advice.

– *Colic*
 • <u>Gastrointestinal</u> : exclude a parasitic infection. Do not give acetylsalicylic acid (possibility of ulcer).
 Depending on severity :
 N-butylhyoscine (PO) :
 Adult : 30-60 mg/d divided in 3 doses x 3-5 days
 or
 atropine (SC) :
 Adult : 0.5 to 1 mg by injection
 Child : 0.01 to 0.02 mg/kg by injection
 • <u>Renal or biliary colic</u> : same as above. If necessary :
 noramidopyrine (IM or IV) :
 Adult : 500 mg by injection

– *Very severe pain*
noramidopyrine (IM or PO)
Adult : 500 mg as necessary
Or, if ineffective :
pentazocine (IM or PO) : 30 mg IM or 50 mg PO as necessary

Fever

Fever is common, and usually, related to an infection of viral, bacterial or parasitic origin. The type and duration of fever helps determine the diagnosis. Note that fever in the newborn has its own complications.

 Fever may be defined as a rectal temperature above 37°C in the morning, and above 37°5C in the evening. The corresponding axillary temperature would be above 37°5C and 38°C. This definition is practical in hospital but not as satisfactory in a dispensary. Several factors have to be considered in taking a patient's temperature : the technique (axillary, oral, rectal), the quality of measurement, the patient compliance, and the time available. One usually considers that axillary temperature under estimates the core temperature by 0°5 C.

– Clinically : any hyperthermia, even if it is only slightly above normal, could be significant (e.g. nocturnal febrile stage in tuberculosis). On the other hand, at dispensary and primary health care level, a higher threshold only should be considered (eg. axillary temperature > 38°C after 5 mins).
At hospital level, a finer thresh-holds can be adopted.
In all cases, **it is essential to define these thresholds**.

– Fever to be treated :
  • In the infant and new born : over 38°C rectal temperature, and / or if there are signs of intolerance.
  • In the adult : above 38°5C and / or if the patient is uncomfortable.

Clinical features

– *The following complications* can be brought about by fever in newborns and infants :
  • Convulsions
  • Dehydration
  • Malignant hyperthermia (collapse and coma)

They should be investigated and treated but moreover they should be prevented (see treatment pages 26-27).

– *Clinical assessment is the main method of investigating the cause of fever.* Epidemiological environment should also be considered. If available, a laboratory could be useful. The following guidelines are helpful. They should be adapted to the epidemiological context, level of medical staff and diagnostic methods.

1

FEVER AS A SERIOUS SYMPTOM OF INFECTION

- High fever, shivering, sweating, malaria endemic area (falciparum), headache, consciousness desorders (even minor) indicate *severe malaria*. Without treatment, it can cause death.Take a malaria smear and treat.
- High fever with general health impairement, with or without other signs indicates *typhoid fever*.
- High fever, stiffness and neurological signs indicate *meningitis* or *meningocephalitis*.
- High fever with :
  - A hemorragical syndrome indicates *meningococcemia*, or *hemorragic fever*, or in an endemic area, *relapsing fever, rickettsiosis, dengue*...
  - Icterus indicates a *hepatitis*...
  - Associated icterus and renal signs (oliguria...) indicates *yellow fever, leptospirosis*...
- Fever with shock indicates *septicemia*.
- Fever with respiratory insufficiency indicates *pneumonia, bronchiolitis, epiglottitis*...
- Fever during last month of pregnancy (major risks to fetus and mother) indicates *falciparum malaria, pyelonephritis*...
- Fever in the new born is always serious.
- Fever in the young adult with general health impairement, adenopathies, chronic diarrhea... indicates a severe *opportunistic infection* in an AIDS patient.

FEVER ASSOCIATED WITH FOCAL SIGNS

Here, diagnosis is easier, for example :
- Pharyngeal signs in *tonsillitis*
- Pulmonary signs in *pneumopathy*
- Cutaneous rash or Koplick spots in *measles*
- Dysentery in *shigellosis*
- Urinary signs in *pyelonephritis*
- Painful swelling of an *abcess* or an *osteomyelitis*...
- Icterus in *hepatitis*...
- Painful large liver in *amœbic abcess*

FEVER WITH NO OBVIOUS FOCAL SIGNS

- Depending on the endemic area and associated clinical picture :
  - *Trypanosomiasis* during blood stage
  - *Bilharzia* during invasive stage
  - *Visceral leishmaniasi*s (Kala-Azar)
  - *Trichinosis* during invasive stage
  - *Brucellosis*
  - *Arbovirus infection* : dengue, scrub typhus...

- Prolonged fever :
  - Tuberculosis, Brucellosis, collagen disease...

"PUO" Pyrexia unknown origin

No sign leads to a diagnosis.
When there is a high rate of PUO, an epidemiological survey is necessary. However, it is recommended to take stock of the situation with the local health authorities, as they have experience of the local conditions and often have the answer to the problem.

Treatment *(dispensary)*

– *Causative* : cause of fever following the established diagnosis of the disease.
– *Symptomatic*
  • Get the patient undressed.
  • Either wet the skin with a tepid sponge (body temperature, not cold) and leave to cool by evaporation, or give a bath at 37°C for a few minutes.
  • Antipyretic treatment (see table 1) :
  paracetamol (PO) :
  Adul : 2 g/d divided in 4 doses
  Child : 30 mg/kg/d divided in 4 doses
  or **acetylsalicylic acid** (**A.S.A.**) (PO) :
  Adult : 3 g/d divided in 3-4 doses
  Child : 50 mg/kg/d divided in 3-4 doses
– Keep the patient well hydrated and breast fed.
– Maintain good nutrition, even if anorexic. Convince the mother to keep feeding.
– With convulsions :
  diazepam : 0,5 mg/kg to be given rectally (use the parenteral solution)
  With diarrhea, give same dose by slow IV injection. Repeat after 10 minutes if necessary (see page 30).

Antipyretic Dosage

Table 1 : *Dosage of acetylsalicylic acid (A.S.A.) and paracetamol by age and weight*

AGE	0	1 month	12 months	5 years	15 years	Adult
WEIGHT	0	4 kg	8 kg	15 kg	35 kg	Adult
A.S.A. tab 500 mg		–	–	3 x 1/4 tab	3 x 1/2 tab	3 x 1 tab
A.S.A. tab 300 mg		–	–	3 x 1/2 tab	3 x 1 tab	3 x 2 tab
A.S.A. tab 75 mg		–	–	3 x 2 tab		
Paracetamol tab 500 mg		–	–	3 x 1/4 tab	3 x 1/2 tab	3 x 1 to 2 tab
Paracetamol tab 100 mg		3 x 1/4 tab	3 x 1/2 tab	3 x 1 tab	3 x 2 tab	

Notes

– **Acetylsalicylic acid (A.S.A.)**

- When used as an anti-inflammatory, the maximum daily dose can be doubled :
  Adult : 6 g
  Child : 100 mg/kg

- In some countries, acetylsalicylic acid is contraindicated in children. Use paracetamol if available.

– **Paracetamol**

- Does not have an anti-inflammatory effect.

- Use in patients with a history of ulcer or gastric problems, in those allergic to acetylsalicylic acid (some asthmatics), in infants and pregnant women.

Anaemia

☞ – Anemia is defined as an abnormally **low concentration of hæmoglobin** in the blood (below 12 g/100ml in males, 11 g/100ml in females). There are three mechanisms : impaired RBC production, RBC loss from bleeding, and increased RBC destruction (hæmolysis).
– Three major causes :
  • **Malaria**
  • **Nutritional deficiencies** in iron and/or folic acid, especially in children and women of childbearing age.
  • **Hookworm**
– Other causes :
  • G6PD deficiency : crisis of hæmolytic anaemia precipitated by certain drugs : chloroquine (perhaps), primaquine, sulfonamides, sulfones, nitrofurans, chloramphenicol, tetracyclines (perhaps), nalidixic acid, acetylsalicylic acid, noramidopyrine, probenecid, niridazole, vitamin K, quinidine...
  • Sickle cell disease, thalassemia
  • Leishmaniasis
  • Bleeding (e.g. gastric ulcer)

Clinical features

– Pallor of conjunctivæ and mucus membranes, fatigue, dizziness, dyspnea, tachycardia, edema, cardiac murmur...
– If possible, determine hemoglobin or hematocrit.
– A blood film will show red cell morphology (but this is difficult to interpret).
– Stool examination to exclude hookworm ; or else in an endemic area treat presumptively with mebendazole.

Treatment

IRON DEFICIENCY ANEMIA *(dispensary)*

ferrous sulphate (PO)
Adult : 0.6 - 1.2 g/d divided in 3 doses x 2 months
Child : 15 to 30 mg/kg/d divided in 3 doses x 2 months

– Often associated with a nutritional deficiency in folate :
folic acid (PO)
Adult : 10-20 mg/d single dose x 15-30 days
Child : 5-15 mg/d single dose x 15-30 days

– Combination tablets can also be used, though the dose of folic acid is low :
ferrous sulphate + folic acid (PO) : as for ferrous sulphate tabs.

– Deworming
mebendazole (PO) : 200 mg in a single dose for all ages.

FOLIC ACID DEFICIENCY *(rarely occurs on its own) (dispensary)*

folic acid (PO)
Adult : 10-20 mg/d single dose x 15-30 days
Child : 5-15 mg/d single dose x 15-30 days

HEMOLYTIC ANEMIA (MALARIA, HÆMOGLOBINOPATHIES) *(dispensary)*

Give **folic acid** only. Do not give iron unless there is a proven associated deficiency (iron from hæmolyzed RBCs remains in the body and is reutilized).

SEVERE ANEMIA WITH SIGNS OF DECOMPENSATION : HÆMATOCRIT LESS THAN 15% OR SIGNS OF CARDIAC FAILURE *(hospital)*

- Transfusion : avoid whenever possible because of risk of transmission of HIV and Hepatitis B viruses. If anaemia is very severe, however, transfusion is life-saving. Use grouped compatible blood ; use packed cells rather than whole blood if possible.
  Volume to be transfused :
  Adult : 2 to 4 bags of packed cells (double volume if whole blood)
  Child : • packed cells : increase in hæmatocrit desired x weight in kg. E.g. 13kg child with Hct of 14% : to bring Hct up to, say, 30%, need to transfuse (30 - 14) x 13 = approx. 200 ml packed cells = approx 400 ml whole blood.
    • whole blood : above volume x 2
    • Rate of transfusion : 2 drops/minute/kg
- Observe very closely (risk of pulmonary edema).

Note : Prevalence of HIV contra-indicates blood transfusion (in the absence of donor blood screening test). Before transfusing measure the risk. Quote : "Transfusions that are not absolutely indicated are contra-indicated".

Prevention

SHORT TERM

- Prophylaxis for pregnant women and malnourished children :
  ferrous sulphate + folic acid (PO)
  Adult : 200 mg + 15-30 mg/d single dose
  Child : 60 mg + 2.5 mg/d single dose
- Dietary Advice

LONG TERM

- Malaria control
- Deworming
- Nutrition education
- Hygiene and sanitation, health and nutritional education, national and local nutrition policy.

Convulsions

☞ – Paroxysmal involuntary movements of cerebral origin with loss of consciousness, often accompanied by biting of the tongue and urinary incontinence.
   – Two priorities :
   • Stop the convulsion.
   • Make an etiological diagnosis quickly and treat the cause. This necessitates a good clinical examination, a blood slide for malaria and possibly a lumbar puncture.

Supportive Treatment

THE PATIENT HAS STOPPED FITTING

– Put in the coma position (lying on left side and upper leg flexed), maintain clear upper airway (remove any secretions or vomitus).
– Treat any fever (see page 26).
– Prepare a syringe of *diazepam* in case of further convulsions.

THE PATIENT IS STILL FITTING

– *diazepam* (IV)
   Adult : 10 mg by slow IV injection (over 2-3 minutes).
   Child : 0.5 mg/kg rectally (use the injectable form) and inject by means of a syringe without a needle, if possible with the help of a nasogastric tube cut to 2-3 cm length. If rectal route impractical because of diarrhea, give same dose by slow IV. If still fitting after 10 minutes, repeat same dose. Child may need to be ventilated if there is respiratory insufficiency secondary to IV diazepam.
   Do not repeat dose if there is no means of ventilation
– Put in coma position, clear out upper airways.
– Treat any fever.

REPEATED GRAND MAL CONVULSIONS

Convulsions which follow each other rapidly or do not cease, carry the risk of respiratory arrest or serious neurological consequences.
– Try *diazepam* 10 mg by slow IV and continue with 40 mg in 500 ml 5 % *glucose* infused over 24 hours. Theoretically, barbiturates IV and assisted ventilation…
– Ensure adequate nutrition and hydration nursing.

REPEATED CONVULSIONS

These can be prevented by oral **phenobarbital** (possibly with gastric tube) or IM if available.
Adult and Child : 3-5 mg/kg/d in 1 or 2 doses without exceeding 200 mg/d.

Injectable phenobarbital must be given through a glass syringe.

Treatment of the Cause

(only causes amenable to treatment are discussed)

INFECTIOUS

- Hyperthermia : treat the fever (see page 26).
- Cerebral malaria (falciparum) (see pages 128-129).
- Meningitis (see page 141).
- Meningo-ncephalitis (e.g. measles, arbovirus) : supportive treatment as for coma :
  feeding-hydration, nursing.

METABOLIC

− Hypoglycemia : may occur in severe malnutrition, neonate or patient being treated
  with IV quinine. Treat with :
  30-50 % solution of **hypertonic glucose** (IV) : 1 g/kg stat followed by 5 % **glucose**
  infusion.

− Hypocalcemia : rickets, malnutrition, neonatal period. Treat with :
  calcium gluconate (ampoule 10 ml = 1 g)
  Adult : 1 g by slow IV injection (= 1 amp)
  Child : 0.04 g/kg by slow IV injection (= 0,4 ml/kg)
  Never use calcium chloride IV.

EPILEPSY

Once commenced, **phenobarbital** treatment must never be abruptly interrupted : risk
of grand mal convulsions. The longer the treatment has lasted, the more gradual it
should be stopped.
In the ambulatory patient, it is often better to leave him with some attacks than risk
abrupt interrumption.

phenobarbital (PO) :
Adult and child : 3-5 mg/kg/d in 1 dose, to be reached gradullay.

If this is insufficient, but only it is available on the spot, the following can be added :
phenytoin (PO) :
Adult : 2-6 mg/kg/d divided in 1-2 doses
Child < 10 years : 3-8 mg/kg/d divided in 1-2 doses
These doses are reached gradually, commencing with 2-3 mg/kg/d in 2 doses. The
same risk with abrupt interrumption.

RECURRENT FEBRILE CONVULSIONS IN CHILDREN

Discuss preventive treatment with diazepam. Avoid phenobarbital.

diazepam (PO) : 0.25 to 0.5 mg/kg/d divided in 3-4 doses

ECLAMPSIA

- *diazepam* : 10 mg slowly IV, plus 40 mg in 500 ml 5 % *glucose* infused over 24 hours.
- Treatment of hypertension : *hydralazine* IV or infusion (see "Hypertension", pages 186-187).
- Obstetrical management (see *"Obstétrique en situation d'isolement"*, Médecins Sans Frontières, 1992).
- Feeding, hydration, nursing.

Shock

 Acute circulatory failure, characterized by a rapid fall in blood pressure which reduces perfusion of the vital organs, causing anoxic damage and preventing the elimination of metabolic waste.

Etiology and Pathophysiology

There are three main mechanisms, more than one may be active in a shocked patient : hypovolæmia, cardiogenic shock, and vasodilatation.

HYPOVOLÆEMIA

– Hemorrhage : trauma, peptic ulcer, ectopic pregnancy, antepartum or postpartum hemorrhage, uterine rupture, etc.
Loss of up to 10-20% of the blood volume may be well tolerated.
Loss of more than 20% of the blood volume does not permit maintenance of adequate blood pressure to perfuse the vital organs.
– Dehydration : prolonged diarrhea and vomiting, cholera, burns, intestinal obstruction, diabetic coma, etc.
– Burns
– Hemolytic crises : malaria, G6PD deficiency and certain medications (see anaemia, page 28).

CARDIOGENIC SHOCK

– Myocardial infarction, terminal congestive cardiac failure.
– Compromised left ventricular filling or emptying : tachyarrythmias, hæmopericardium, pericardial tamponade, tension pneumothorax, massive pulmonary embolism.

VASODILATATION

– Septic shock : septicemia, release of bacterial endotoxins.
– Anaphylactic shock : release of histamine and other vasodilators.

Clinical features

HYPOVOLEMIC OR CARDIOGENIC SHOCK

– Patient usually conscious, but apathetic.
– Palor, marbled skin, cold and clammy extremities.
– Rapid thready pulse (rate >120), blood pressure low or undetectable.
– Rapid breathing.
– Oliguria or anuria.

Septic shock

- Early : fever, chills, warm extremities.
- Rapid pulse, variable BP.
- Hyperventilation.

Signs related to specific etiologies

- Loss of skin elasticity : dehydration.
- Chest pain : infarction, pulmonary embolism.
- Abdominal guarding : peritonitis, distension due to obstruction.
- Melaena : GIT hemorrhage.

Management (hospital)

- Lie patient down, keep warm, elevate legs.
- Establish IV line : large vein, large bore needle (16 or 18G for adult).
- Cardiac arrest : external cardiac massage.
- Respiratory arrest : endotracheal intubation, manual ventilation.
- Close monitoring of vital signs : pulse, BP, respiratory rate, urine output.

Treatment of the cause (hospital)

Hypovolemia

- *Hemorrhage*
  Rapid transfusion of as many units of crossmatched blood (which has been HIV tested) has necessary to maintain a stable blood pressure. Meanwhile, prepare to surgically treat the cause of the hemorrhage.
  <u>Note</u> : the absence of HIV testing, refer to note on page 29.

- *Acute dehydration*
  Infusion of **Plasmion**® or **Haemacel**® : 1 to 2 bottles (child : 10 to 20 mg/kg), given in a jet thann :
  ringer lactate solution
  Adult and child : 100 ml/kg over 4 hours, then 100 ml/kg in the next 20 hours.

Cardiogenic shock

- *Cardiac failure and acute pulmonary edema*
  - half-sitting position, legs lower than body.
  - **furosemide** : 40 to 80 mg IV stat. Higher doses sometimes needed. Observe pulse, BP and urine output.
  - **digoxin** (only if no cardiac arrythmia) :
    Adult : 0.25 mg IV stat
    Child : 0.01 mg/kg IV stat

1

- Beri-Beri may be a cause of cardiac failure. Treat with
  Thiamine (IM) :
  Adult : 200 mg IM or IV /d
  Child : 50 - 100 mg IM or IV /d   for a few days then PO
- If furosemide not available, rapid blood letting through basilar vein (300-400 ml in the absence of a severe anaemia) in severe cases.

– *Tamponade* (due to acute constrictive pericarditis, often tuberculous)
  Requires urgent pericardial tap.

– *Myocardial infarction* : rare in tropical countries.
  - Treat the pain with **pentazocine** : 30 mg IM.
  - Nitrite derivatives if available.

– *Tension pneumothorax* : <u>urgent pleural aspiration</u>.

VASODILATATION

– *Septic shock*
  - Find the focus of infection : abscess, RTI, digestive system, gynaecology).
  - Antibiotics :
    ampicillin : 100 to 200 mg/kg/24 hours, divided in 3-4 IV injections/24 hours
  - Plus, if available :
    gentamicin : 3 mg/kg/24 hours, IM, without exceeding 180 mg/24 hours or 3 IM injections/24 hours
  - Controversial : corticosteroids.

– *Anaphylactic shock*
  Determine and remove the cause (e.g. insect sting, drug).
  epinephrin (adrenaline) :
  Adult : 0.5 to 1 mg diluted in 10 ml isotonic solution (glucose, normal saline, ringer lactate) by slow IV infusion.
  Child : 0.25 mg diluted in 10 ml isotonic solution (glucose, normal saline, ringer lactate) by slow IV infusion.

Note that the management of a shocked patient must always include very close monitoring of vital signs and clinical progress. All parameters should be noted on an observation form.

Severe protein-energy malnutrition

Malnutrition occurs because of a prolonged discrepancy between food consumption and nutritional needs.

To understand malnutrition requires first a knowledge of the prevalence in the childhood population and second a study of the individual causes (pathology, weaning problems) or collective causes (famine, drought, economic problems) in order to determine appropriate treatment measures.

How to determine nutritional state

CLINICAL SIGNS

Marasmus	*Kwashiorkor*	*Maras-Kwashiorkor*
Muscle wasting and loss of sub-cutaneous tissue. Loss of appetite Reduced growth Irritability	Weight loss, Œdema of extremities (and the face) Loss of appetite Skin changes Apathy Changes of the hair and nails	Two classes of signs : muscle wasting and œdema

CLASSIFICATION

There are several types of classification. It is helpfull to use anthropometric measurements to determine the severity of the malnutrition.

The most frequently used indicators are :

– *Classification of weight/age*

Weight of the subject / Normal weight of a child of the same age.
80 - 60 % : moderate malnutrition
< 60 %   : severe malnutrition

– *Classification of weight/height*

Weight of the subject / Normal weight of a child of the same height.
80 - 70 % : moderate malnutrition
< 70 %   : severe malnutrition

– *Arm circumference*

Measure the arm circumference in the middle of the upper arm of a child aged 1 to 5 years.

13,5 cm - 12,5 cm : moderate malnutrition
< 12 cm : severe malnutrition

– *Presence of tibial œdema*

This indicates severe malnutrition.

Beyond their use to study the prevalence of malnutrition in the population, anthropometric indicators establish the criteria for entry to and exit from the feeding center.

Example (weight/height) :
- criteria for entry = < 70 % W/H
- criteria for exit = > 85 % W/H for two consecutive measurements, improving general state and disappearing œdema.

Different types of treatment

FEEDING CENTER FOR THE SEVERELY MALNOURISHED

First establish a system adapted to needs which depends on the number of cases : establish a specific structure = center of therapeutic recuperation (intensive), or indeed a pediatric service if the numbers are not too large.

Treatment continues on a 24 hour cycle 7 days a week. The treatment center is essential and depends on the active participation of the mothers under the supervision of trained personnel. A medical center is indispensable.

The principle of treating the malnourished persons is to progressively give calories and protein at appropriate stages of treatment :

– *Acute phase*
- reanimation and initiation of dietary cure
- maintenance

– *Recuperation phase*
- enhanced growth
- return to family meals

ACUTE PHASE

– **Reanimation and initiation of dietary cure**

Reanimation is the medical treatment of the complications of malnutrition, in particular dehydration.

Initiation of a cure leads at the same time to reanimation.

Nutrition must be progressive and not agressive. Give small frequent meals because these reduce the risk of diarrhea, vomiting, hypoglycemia and hypothermia. Always adapt treatment to the individual.

Infants are given oral nourishment (by spoon, never by bottle) or by nasogastric tube if anorexic or there is severe vomiting.

The regime should be max 80 to 100 Kcal/kg body weight in the first days with a minimum of protein.

– *Maintenance*

A phase of stabilisation occurs during treatment : at the stage, attempts should be made to "recuperate" the weight lost.

Note a reduction of the œdema or stagnation in kwashiorkor.

This phase continues until the appetite returns.

If the child is still being breast fed, it is necessary to continue and encourage this method of nutrition.

The following protocol can be used for example :

20 g (45 ml) DSM (dry skimmed milk)	reconstitute with 1 liter of water :
100 g (100 ml) sugar	
40 g (40 ml) oil	100 Kcal and 0.6 g of protein/100 ml

Treatment of acute phase	Number of meal/day	Volume of meal (ml/kg)	Protein g/kg/day	Energy Kcal/kg/day
Initiation				
Day 1 and 2	12	10	0.6	100
Day 3 to 5	8	15	0.6	100
Maintenance Stating on the 6th day	6	20	0.6	100

Meals are given every two hours. Gorging of food can be used, this is practiced on day 1 and 2, under the surveillance of a nurse or other health worker.

The acute phase lasts for 7 days with marasmus. For a child with œdema, the progression from initial treatment to cure must be slow and the maintenance phase prolonged. The œdema decreases and the general state improves with the stage of rehabilitation (about 15 days).

1

RECUPERATION PHASE

– **Enhanced growth**

The objective is to achieve no more weight for height as quickly as possible.

The speed of weight gain is directly proportional to alimentary consumption. Minimal requirement corresponds to 150-200 Kcal/kg/day and 4 to 5 g of protein/kg/day.

The principle occupation at the stage is to institute concentrated high energy alimentation because a child of less than 5 years only absorbs illimited amount.

Use high energy concentrated alimentation : oil, sugar... and continue to give as many small meals as possible per day.

A possible formula for high energy alimentation is :

90 g (200 ml) DSM
60 g (60 ml)   sugar
80 g (80 ml)   oil   1000 ml
        800 ml   water

128 Kcal and 3.2 g of protein/100 ml
192 Kcal and 4.8 g of protein/100 ml

Many of the formulas are available, notably that of Oxfam :

6 volumes of powder milk
2 volumes of oil   premix
1 volume of sugar

premix = dry mixture
H.E.M. = premix + water (H.E.M. = high energy milk)

1 volume of premix + 4 volumes of water —> H.E.M.
100 ml of H.E.M. = 100 Kcal + 4 g of protein (1 ml = 1 Kcal)

– **Return to family meals**

The move to family meals is an important step in recuperation.

Meals should be introduced progressively. Insist on the importance of the participation of mothers and their education in nutrition.

Medical feeding center

ASSOCIATED PATHOLOGIES

The associated pathologies must be treated :

– Diarrhea :
  ORS (see pages 82-83)

- Bacterial infections
  antibiotics

- Buccal candidiasis
  gentian violet

- Intestinal parasites
  mebendazole : 200 mg/d x 3 days

- Anti-malaria prophylaxis
  chloroquine : 10 mg/kg/week

- Skin lesions
  zinc oxide ointment

- Look for tuberculosis
  Tuberculosis should always be suspected if, after several weeks of treatment, a
  child is not recovering.

SPECIFIC NUTRIENT DEFICIENCIES

These should be corrected if possible :

- **Potassium** : 5 mmol/kg/day

- **Magnesium** : 2 mmol/kg/day

- **Zinc** : 2 mg/kg/day

- Multivitamin preparation and **vitamin C** (see page 76)

- **Vitamin A** : according to WHO recommendations

- **Iron** : from the reanimation phase (see page 29)

- **Folic acid** : 5 mg/day

FLUID REQUIREMENTS

- It is important to give water to the malnourished infant, several times a day,
  between meals, especially if the outside temperature is high, or if the infant has a
  fever, and educate the mother to this effect.

- It is necessary however to use ORS with discrimination : only if there is diarrhea
  and, if it is poorly tolerated, cut the volume to 1/2 or 1/3.

Surveillance

Pay particular attention to the changing state of each case, in particular by following
the weight gain and by medical examination. All personnel in the feeding center
must be able to analyse cases and act appropriatly.

This surveillance must be organised :

– Control the allocation of meals and their preparation.

– Regularly gather information : register weight (especially during acute phase).

– Repeated medical consultations, register medications.

1

CHAPTER 2

Respiratory diseases

2

Strategy for the control of acute respiratory infections in developing countries

2

In developing countries, lower respiratory tract infections are one of the main causes of mortality in children under 5 years of age. A large proportion of these infections are bacterial. Prompt treatment with an appropriate antibiotic will therefore assist in decreasing child mortality.

At the peripheral dispensary level, simple, reliable clinical criteria are needed to allow health workers to decide whether :
– to give antibiotics for moderate cases ;
– to refer severe cases to a doctor or hospital.

This chapter is based upon the WHO (38) strategy which aims to define these criteria. This chapter only deals with lower respiratory tract infections.

Management of the child with a cough

Cough is always present in upper or lower respiratory tract infections (rare exceptions). Diagnosis and treatment are based on cough.

WHEN DOES A CHILD WITH A COUGH NEED ANTIBIOTIC TREATMENT ?

Most of coughing children do not need antibiotics. But association of cough and some other signs indicates that A.R.I. should be treated with antibiotics.

– *Positive criteria*
   If one or several of those following criteria exist, antibiotic treatment :
   • Tachypnea > 50 respirations/minute
   • Alar flare (dilatation of the nostrils with each inspiration)
   • Chest indrawing (sternal or intercostal recession)
   • Cyanosis
   • Child unable to drink
   • Child malnourished (< 70% weight-for-height or kwashiorkor)
   • Post-measles

– *Criteria that are not useful at a dispensary level*
   • Fever (since viral infections also cause fever)
   • Yellow sputum (difficult symptom to assess in a young child)
   • Chest auscultation (needs a doctor, difficult in tiny children)

WHEN SHOULD A CHILD BE REFERRED TO HOSPITAL ?

Although tachypnea is the best predictor of the presence of pneumonia, the severity is best judged by chest indrawing.
- Chest indrawing (sternal or intercostal recession), except if child is less than 1 month of age or child has asthma, as in these two conditions chest indrawing can be present even with mild disease. In these cases, use tachypnea as the main criterion.
- Tachypnea > 60 respirations / minute.
- Cyanosis.
- Child unable to drink.
- Respiratory fatigue or apnœic periods.
- Clouded consciousness.
- Stridor
- Convulsions

WHICH ANTIBIOTIC SHOULD BE CHOSEN TO TREAT PNEUMONIA IN A CHILD UNDER 5 YEARS OF AGE ?

Account should be taken of bacterial activity, effectiveness, ease of availibility (price, supplies...) and side effects.

Dispensary : according to the situation and to availability, the choice should be made from the following four antibiotics :
1. *cotrimoxazole* per os : 40 mg/kg/d of SMX divided in 2 doses
2. *amoxycillin* per os : 50 mg/kg/d divided in 3 doses
3. *ampicillin* per os : 100 mg/kg/ddivided in 3 doses   x 5 days
4. *PPF* IM : 50,000 to 100,000 IU/kg once daily
   (or *procain penicillin*)   avoid in children less than 1 year of age
5. *chloramphenicol* per os : 50 to 75 mg/kg/d divided in 3 doses

Choice is determined by the national recommendations of the country.

Hospital : the same antibiotics as above. Two special situations:

- *Serious cases, or need for parenteral administration*
  ampicillin (IM - IV) : 100 mg/kg/d divided in 3 injections / 24 hours
  chloramphenicol (IM - IV) : 50 to 75 mg/kg/d divided in 3 injections / 24 hours
  Treat for 7 days. If possible, switch to oral forms after 72 hours.

- *Neonatal pneumonia*
  ampicillin IV : 100 mg/kg/d divided in 3 injections x 7 days
  Depending on gravity, combine this with:
  gentamicin IM : < 10 days : 4 mg/kg/d divided in 2 injections x 7 days
                    10 days to 1 year : 6 mg/kg/d divided in 2-3 injections x 7 days

Note : in situations where the patient will only be seen once (such as mobile clinics, or with nomads), one can use a slow-release depot preparation, *oil chloramphenicol* : 100 mg/kg in 1 IM injection, repeated after 48 hours if possible.

Table 2 : *Comparison of different antibiotics used to treat respiratory infections*

Antibiotics	Spectrum (main pathogens)	Cost FF* Child 10 kg / 5 days	Side effects	Ease of use Number of doses/day
ORAL				
Penicillin V	Pneumococcus	1.25	Penicillin allergy	3 doses/d
Ampicillin or *Amoxycillin*	Pneumococcus Hæm. Influenzae Gram – bacilli	3.60 2.50	Penicillin allergy	3 doses/d 3 doses/d
Cotrimoxazole	Pneumococcus Hæm. Influenzae Staphylocoque aureus Chlamydia Pneumocystis	0.50	Rare but may be fatal : Stevens-Johnson synd. Contraindicated in infants < 2 months	2 doses/d
Erythromycin	Chlamydia Mycoplasma Pneumococcus	3.00	Few : GIT	3 doses/d
Chloramphenicol	Hæm. Influenzae Pneumococcus Staphylo. aureus Gram – bacilli	1.35	Agranulocytosis grey syndrome (rare but serious) Contraindicated in infant < 2 mth	3 doses/d
Tetracyclines	Hæm. Influenzae Pneumococcus Chlamydia Mycoplasma	0.60	GIT : staining of teeth and bones Contraindicated in children < 8 years and pregn.	3 doses/d
IM / IV				
Benzyl Peni	In adequat dosage, active against Pneumococcus	34.00	Penicillin allergy	4 inj./d
PPF or *Procain Peni*	Hæm. Influenzae	2.50		1 inj./d
Ampicillin or *Amoxycillin*	as above	12.30	Penicillin allergy	3 inj./d
Chloramphenicol	as above	8.00	Agranulocytosis	3 inj./d
Gentamicin	Gram – Staphylocci	1.00	Nephrotoxic ototoxic	2 to 3 inj./d

* Average price of generic drug in 1988.

SUPPORTIVE THERAPY

– Oxygen
  • Expensive, difficult to procure, questionable effectiveness.
  • Reserve for cyanosed asthmatic children or those with RR > 70.
  • Administer by intranasal catheter, flow rate 1 litre/min.
– Food and fluids
  • Imperative to continue breast feeding.
  • Encourage oral fluids ; use nasogastric tube if necessary.
  • Encourage child to eat.
– Keep nose clear
  • Lavage with syringe and *normal saline* (Nacl 0.9 % or ringer lactate) in hospital.
  • Show mother how to use a clean piece of cloth at home.
– Temperature
  • Treat any fever above 38°C (see pages 26-27).
  • Treat for malaria in an endemic zone (see pages 128-129).
– Humidify air : If possible : wet sheet across top of cot...
– Do not give antitussive medicines : expensive and sometimes dangerous.

MANAGEMENT BY A HEALTH AUXILLARY OF UNDER-FIVES WITH LOWER RESPIRATORY TRACT INFECTIONS

(the health auxillary should have received at least 6 months training)

– When an antibiotic is needed it should be given as early in the illness as possible.
– The auxillary must be able to decide properly when to refer to hospital.

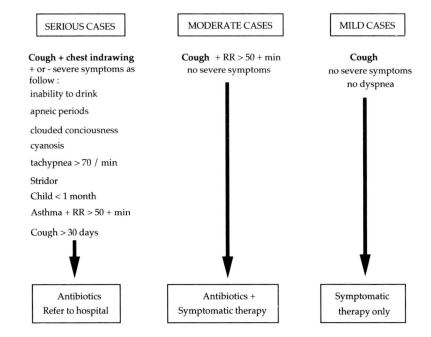

SERIOUS CASES	MODERATE CASES	MILD CASES
Cough + chest indrawing + or - severe symptoms as follow :	**Cough** + RR > 50 + min no severe symptoms	**Cough** no severe symptoms no dyspnea
inability to drink		
apneic periods		
clouded conciousness		
cyanosis		
tachypnea > 70 / min		
Stridor		
Child < 1 month		
Asthma + RR > 50 + min		
Cough > 30 days		
Antibiotics Refer to hospital	Antibiotics + Symptomatic therapy	Symptomatic therapy only

Some upper respiratory tract infections require antibiotic treatment :

- Acute laryngitis : because of the severe dyspnea, this condition will be classified as a serious case and will receive antibiotics.

- Tonsillitis et otitis media : cough is often associated for antibiotic indication refer to pages 51-54.

2

MEASURES FOR PRESENTING LOWER RESPIRATORY TRACT INFECTIONS IN THE UNDER-FIVES

- Improve environment (better housing, less crowding).

- Bedding, blankets, clothing.

- Better nutrition.

- Immunization against measles, pertussis and diphtheria : Expanded Program of Immunization (EPI).

Common cold

 Viral infection of the nasopharyngeal mucosa which are frequent and seasonal. Person to person transmission is usually airborne.

Clinical features

– Runny nose, often with fever and cough.

– May be the prodrome of influenza or measles.

– Sometimes accompanied by conjunctivitis.

Treatment (dispensary)

– Nasopharyngeal lavage using a syringe filled with **normal saline** (or clean water with **ORS** added, 1 sachet/litre), 4 to 6 times a day.

– Treat fever (see pages 26-27).

– Treat or take preventive steps against conjunctivitis (see pages 105-106).

– If allergic component (morning sneezing fits) :
promethazine (PO)
Adult : 75 mg/d divided in 3 doses x 3-5 days
Child : 1 mg/kg/d divided in 3 doses x 3-5 days
or
chlorphenamine : 12 mg/d divided in 3 doses x 3-5 days

Follow-up

Risk of secondary infection and acute otitis media in infants. Always check the tympanic membranes of an infant with a cold.

Pharyngitis and Tonsillitis

2

☞ Infection and inflammation of the pharynx and tonsils accompanied by fever, dysphagia and adenopathy.

Treatment

The two main objectives of therapy are to recognise and treat the tonsillitis of diphtheria and to reduce the complications of streptococcal throat infections (acute rheumatic fever and cardiac lesions).

Table 3 : *Etiology and treatment of pharyngitis and tonsillitis according to appearance of the throat*

Throat & Tonsils	Other signs	Likely cause	Treatment
Red ± exudate *(dispensary)*	Fever ++ Dysphagia ++	After 3 years : Streptococcal	After 3 years : *Peni V* Ad. : 1.5 to 3 MIU in 3 doses x 7 d Child : 50,000 U/kg/d in 3 doses x 7 d
			If allergic : *Erythromycin* per os Ad. : 1 g/d divided in 3 doses x 7 d Child: 50 mg/kg/d x 7 d
		Before 3 years : Viral, sometimes streptococcal-	Before 3 years : Treat severe cases or those with adeno- pathy as above
Ulcerated necrotic *(dispensary)*		Fusospirochaetes (Vincent's bacilli)	*Penicillin* or If allergic : *Erythromycin*
False membranes (grey, adhere to mucosa, extensive) *(hospital)* *(hospital)*	Alterated general state, Croup Cardiac signs Unimmunized ...	Diphtheria	*PPF* IM : 100,000 U/kg/d x 7 d *Serotherapy* IM (equine antitoxin) Adult : 60 -120,000 U Child : 30 - 60,000 U

– Always treat the fever and keep well hydrated (dysphagia).

– Patients with infectious mononucleosis will almost always present with an allergy to ampicillin. Stop the treatment.

– Follow-up to exclude acute rheumatic fever (polyarthritis, cardiac signs) and glomerulonephritis (edema, proteinuria, hypertension, hematuria).

– In case of diphteria, procede a survey in the patient neighbourhood. Contacts should be systematically treated with **penicillin** or **erythromycin**.

Note

Test the sensitivity to the equine antitoxin (SC 0.1 ml), wait 20 minutes to check an adverse reaction before complete treatment.

Acute otitis

Otitis externa

 Infection of external auditory meatus (sometimes due to a foreign body).

Clinical features

- Pain, elicited especially by traction upon the pinna.
- Redness of meatus + abscess.
- May be an exudate.
- Drum normal.

Treatment (dispensary)

- Analgesia : *acetylsalicylic acid* or *paracetamol* (see page 27).
- Local : if exudate lavage with *normal saline*. Apply *gentian violet* with a cotton bud for 3-5 days.
- If present, remove the foreign body.

Otitis media

 Acute infection of the middle ear. Usually bacterial, tracking up from the nasopharynx : streptococcal, pneumococcal, Hemophilus influenzae in children under 5 years.

Clinical features

- Fever, severe pain, crying, agitation, vomiting, diarrhea.
- Ear drum : becomes progressively congested, inflamed, bulging, and finally perforates with release of pus.

Treatment *(dispensary)*

– Treat for fever and pain (see pages 26-27).

– If upper respiratory tract infection : nasopharyngeal lavage (ringer lactate).

– Rehydration if necessary.

– Antibiotherapy :

- *Over 5 years*
  Adult : *penicillin V*(PO) : 2 MIU/d divided in 3 doses x 10 days
  Child : *penicillin V*(PO) : 100,000 IU /kg/d divided in 3 doses x 10 days
           or
           PPF (ou *procain penicillin*) : 100,000 IU/kg/d IM x 3 days, then *peni V* per
           os : same dose divided in 3 doses/day (total treatment : 10 days)
  If allergic to penicillin :
  erythromycin (PO) :
  Adult : 1.5-2 g/d divided in 3 doses x 10 days
  Child : 50 mg/kg/d divided in 3 doses x 10 days

- *Under 5 years*
  ampicillin (PO) : 100 mg/kg/d divided in 3 doses x 10 days
  or
  cotrimoxazole (PO) : 60 mg/kg/d SMX divided in 2 doses x 10 days

– Paracentesis : is indicated if the ear drum is bulging but not yet perforated. Should be done in the infero-posterior quadrant. Aspirate the pus and prescribe an antibiotic as above.

Prognosis

If neglected, acute otitis media may become chronic. There is also a risk of mastoiditis.

Chronic otitis

☞ Chronic infection of the middle ear with perforation of the tympanic membrane.

Clinical features

– Chronic discharge (otorrhea)
– Occasional acute re-infection : fever + pain, usually associated with an obstruction to drainage through the perforated drum with secondary infection by streptococci, pneumococci or gram negative organisms.

Treatment (dispensary)

– Do not prescribe antibiotics.
– Only if acute re-infection occurs give :
  ampicillin
  or
  cotrimoxazole
  in the same doses as for acute otitis media.
  Lavage with *normal saline* and aspirate with a syringe.
– Always put a little dry cotton wool or small wick in the ear to absorb the discharge ; change 3-4 times/day til dried up.

Prognosis

– Risk of deafness in affected ear.
– Risk of mastoiditis and meningitis during acute re-infections.

Acute laryngitis

 Acute infections of the laryngeal mucosa often associated with viral infections (e.g. colds, measles...).

Prognosis

The prognosis is good. However, patients sometimes develop partial respiratory obstruction, and it is important to identify these "high risk" situations and to take the necessary precautions.

ADULT

– Usually associated with a "hoarse" voice and a cold. The etiology is viral.
  Symptomatic treatment : *A.A.S.* or *paracetamol* (PO) (see page 27).

– Rarely, epiglottitis from H. influenzae, diphtheria or retropharyngeal abscess. In these cases, use the same methods as for treating children.

– Tuberculous laryngitis.

CHILD

There is a risk of respiratory obstruction.

Signs of distress

Inspiratory stridor, with or without intercostal recession, pallor, with or without cyanosis with cough and "croupy" voice.
There are 2 distinct clinical features.

1. *Progressive dyspnea* (1 or more days)

In a child < 3 years, if other causes have been eliminated (e.g. diphtheria, retropharyngeal abscess, foreign body), the dyspnea is probably due to mild subglottic obstruction from a viral infection (laryngo-tracheobronchitis).
It is important to watch the child carefully, to keep him calm and to provide humidified air.
Antibiotics are unnecessary except for secondary infections (use PO *ampicillin* or *cotrimoxazole*). Steroids are not useful.
If the dyspnea worsens, intubation or tracheostomy may be necessary.

2. *Rapid onset dyspnea* (several hours)

Carefully examine the patient in a sitting position. <u>Do not lie them down</u>.

– *Foreign body* : if the dyspnea becomes labored, remove foreign body rapidly, in surgical surroundings.

– *Acute epiglottitis from Hæmophilus influenzae*
  • Child of 3 - 8 years : sudden onset dyspnea, high fever, stridor, dysphagia (drools saliva), breathes through mouth, cervical lymphadenopathy.
  • Do not lie the patient down and avoid examining the larynx as these actions may precipitate respiratory obstruction.
  • Keep the child sitting in a humid atmosphere. Give :
    ampicillin (IV) : 200 mg/kg/24 hours divided in 3-4 injections, reverting to oral treatment as soon as possible ; total duration : 7 days
    or
    chloramphenicol (IV) : 100 mg/kg/d divided in 3-4 injections, reverting to oral treatment as soon as possible ; total duration : 7 days
  • Severe distress or obstruction : tracheostomy.

– *Recurrent laryngitis*
  • Child of 2-4 years with a cold or measles.
  • Nocturnal dyspnea with no fever.
  • Place the infant in humidified atmosphere.
  • Eventually, give :
    promethazine (PO) : 75 mg/kg/d divided in 3 doses x 5 days
    or
    chlorphenamine (PO) : 12 mg/d divided in 3 doses x 5 days

– *Diphtheria* : false membrane in the throat
  • Unvaccinated children.
  • Sometimes the false membrane is extensive an adherent.
  • Poor general condition.
  • Treatment (see page 51) :
    diphtheria antitoxin
    penicillin G or ***PPF*** IM
  • Tracheostomy if necessary.

Sinusitis

☞ Infection of the sinus mucosæ with purulent nasal discharge. May originate from :

– the nose : rhinitis, allergic rhinitis, nasal obstruction (e.g. mal-formation, trauma) ;

– the teeth : caries with arthritis and / or osteitis.

Clinical features

Associated with **pain** and a **purulent nasal discharge**.

ADULT

– Pain
  • Periorbital : frontal sinusitis.
  • Facial : maxillary or ethmoidal sinusitis.

– Purulent unilateral nasal discharge on the affected side with nasal obstruction and a moderate fever.

– Examination :
  • Exquisite tenderness can be elicited over these points.
  • Rhinoscopy : inflamed mucosa with purulent exudate.

Bacteria responsible are Hæmophilus influenzae in persons < 5 years and pneumococcus in older persons.

INFANTS

Acute ethmoiditis : high fever, edema of lower eyelids and the bridge of the nose with purulent rhinorrhea.

Danger of spread to bone or orbit. Treat vigorously.

Bacteria responsible are Hæmophilus, pneumococcus and staphylococcus.

2

Treatment *(dispensary)*

– Nasopharyngeal lavage (see page 50) with removal of foreign body (if found).

– **A.A.S.** or **paracetamol** for fever and pain (see pages 26-27).

– If dental focus of infection, extract tooth under antibiotic cover.

– Antibiotic :
cotrimoxazole (PO) : 60 mg of SMX/kg/d divided in 2 doses x 10 days
or
ampicillin (PO) : 100 mg/kg/d divided in 3 doses x 10 days

– *Ethmoiditis*
ampicillin (IV) : 200 mg/kg/d divided in 3 or 4 injections stat until cured. Change to PO as soon as possible.
or
chloramphenicol (IV or IM) : 100 mg/kg/d divided in 3 or 4 injections, then change to PO as soon as possible.

Prognosis

Acute sinusitis may become chronic, so always exclude other pathology (e.g. foreign body, allergy, dental caries...).

Bronchitis

Acute bronchitis

 Acute infection of the bronchial mucosa.

Clinical features

- Often preceded by an upper respiratory tract infection.
- Cough, dry at first, then productive.
- Low grade fever.
- No marked dyspnea.
- Scattered rhonchi.

Treatment (dispensary)

- In basically healthy patient following *rhino-pharyngitis* or *flu*.
  - Keep well hydrated, treat fever, humidified air if possible.
  - Nasopharyngeal lavage with *isotonic solution* (normal saline or ringer lactate).
  - No antibiotics (mostly viral).

- In patient with poor basic health (malnutrition, measles, rickets, anaemia, chronic bronchitis, cardiac disease, elderly...) or dyspnea > 50 mn or other serious signs (see page 48).

  In these cases, superinfection is probable (haemophilus, gram -- bacilli, pneumococcus). Treat with :
  cotrimoxazole (PO)
  Adult : 1,600 mg/d of SMX divided in 2 doses x 5-7 days
  Child : 60 mg/kg/d of SMX divided in 2 doses x 5-7 days

  or
  ampicillin (PO) : 100 mg/kg/d divided in 3 doses x 5-7 days

  or
  chloramphenicol (PO) : 50 mg/kg/d divided in 3 doses x 5-7 days

- Where wheezing occurs, treat as asthma (see page 67).

Chroniques

☞ Chronic inflammation of the bronchial mucosa of irritant (tobacco) or allergic (asthma) origin, progressing towards chronic respiratory failure.
Part of the syndrome of chronic obstructive airways disease (COAD).

2

Clinical features

- Morning cough, clear sputum, bronchial rales.

- If secondary infection : fever and purulent sputum.

- Always exclude TB : sputum smear for AFB.

Treatment (dispensary)

- Discourage cigarette smoking.

- No antibiotics unless secondary infection. In this case, see acute bronchitis.

Pneumonia and Bronchopneumonia

 Infection of pulmonary alveoli and bronchial mucosa.
Cause :
- viral
- bacterial : pneumococcus, Hæmophilus influenzæ, mycoplasma pneumonia
- parasitic : pneumocystis carinii (AIDS)

Clinical features

- High fever (> 39°), cough, respiratory distress, chest pain and tachypnea (> 50/min).
- Examination : dullness to percussion, diminished vesicular breath sounds, crepitations and sometimes bronchial breath sounds.

Treatment

Depends on age and presence of respiratory distress tachypnea (> 60/mn in infants less than 2 months, > 50/mn from 2 to 12 months, > 40/mn from 1 to 5 years), intercostal recession, alar flare, stridor, cyanosis, respiratory pauses, xyphi-sternal recession.
Other serious extrapulmonary signs can be present (see pages 45-46).

ABSENCE OF SERIOUS SIGNS

- *Classical pneumonia in adults and children < 5 years*

Localised crepitation, sometimes bronchial breathing or localised dullness to percussion = pneumococcus. By far the most common germ after 5 years of age.

Treatment (dispensary)
penicillin V(PO) :
Adult : 2,4-3,6 MIU/d divided in 3 doses (tab 250 mg = 0.4 MIU : 2-3 tab x 3/d) x 5 days
Child : 50 000 IU/kg/divided in 3 doses x 5 days
or
cotrimozazole (PO) :
Adult : 1600 mg of SMX/divided in 2 doses x 5 days
Child : 50 mg of SMX/kg/divided in 2 doses x 5 days

– *Pneumonia in child of 2 months to 5 years*

H. Influenzae common at this age. Therefore, first line of treatment :
cotrimoxazole (PO) : 50 mg of SMX/kg/d divided in 2-3 doses x 5 days
or
ampicillin (PO) : 100 mg/kg/d divided in 3-4 doses x 5 days
or
amoxycillin (PO) : 50 mg/kg/d divided in 3 doses x 5 days, depending on availability

– *Pneumonia in infant < 2 months*

Hospitalize (risk of rapid decompensation).
ampicillin PO if possible (if not IM) : 100 mg/kg/d divided in 3-4 doses x 7 days

Always treat fever and ensure adequate hydration and nourishment. Always review the patient 2 days later.

PNEUMONIA WITH RESPIRATORY DISTRESS : HOSPITALIZE

– *Adult and child > 5 years*

• If clinical evidence favours pneumococcus (one or several systematic foci with crepitation and/or decreased vesicular breath sounds, sometimes bronchial breathing or dullness to percussion) :
PPF IM :
Adult : 3-4 MIU/d in 1 injection x 2-3 days
          then commence oral therapy with *peni V* : 3-4 MIU/d divided in 3-4 doses to complete 7 days
Child : 50.000 UI/kg/d in 1 dose x 2-3 days
          then commence oral therapy with *péni V*: 50.000 IU/kg/d divided in 3-4 doses to complete 7 days
or
chloramphenicol IV-IM :
Adult : 3-4 g/d divided in 3-4 doses over several days, then commence orally (same dosage) to complete 7 days
Child : 100 mg/kg/d divided in 3-4 doses over several days, then commence orally (same dosage) to complete 7 days

• In all other cases :
chloramphenicol IV or IM :
Adult : 3-4 g/d divided in 3-4 doses over 2-3 days
Child : 100 mg/kg/d divided in 3-4 doses over 2-3 days, then in both cases change to oral treatment with the same dosage to complete 7 days
or
ampicillin IV or IM :
Adult : 3-4 g/d divided in 3-4 doses over 2-3 days
Child : 100 mg/kg/d divided in 3-4 doses over 2-3 days, then in both cases change to oral treatment with the same dosage to complete 7 days

Where no improvement with ampicillin after 2 days, combine with
gentamicin IM :
Adult : 160 mg/d divided in 2 doses
Child : 3-6 mg/kg/d divided in 2 doses x 7 days

– *Child of 2 months to 5 years*

chloramphenicol IV or IM : 100 mg/kg/d divided in 3-4 doses ; change to oral treatment as soon as possible in the same dosage to complete 7-10 days
or
ampicillin IV or IM : 100 mg/kg/d divided in 3-4 doses ; change to oral treatment as soon as possible in the same dosage to complete 7-10 days
When possible, combine with *gentamicin* IM : 6 mg/kg/d divided in 2 doses during 7-10 days

In the absence of improvement or when deterioration occurs at the end of properly conducted treatment, think about staphylococcal pneumonia (see page 65).

– *Infant < 2 months*

ampicillin IV o IM : 100 mg/kg/d divided in 3-4 doses ; change to oral treatment as soon as possible in the same dosage to complete 7-10 days
plus *gentamicin* IM : 6 mg/kg/d divided in 2-3 doses x 7-10 days (for neonates < 10 days old : 4 mg/kg/d in 2 doses))

When no improvement occurs or there is deterioration after 4 days of correct treatment, think about a staphylococcal pneumonia (see "staphylococcal pneumonia", page 65).

In all cases, treat the temperature, ensure adequate nutrition and hydration (gastric tube if necessary). If oxygen available, use by means of nasal tube at the rate of 1 litre per minute when there is respiratory distress.

REFRACTORY PNEUMONIA IN ADULTS OR OLDER CHILDREN

Consider atypical pneumonia (mycoplasma) or tuberculosis. Alternative therapies to try :
tetracycline
Adult   : 1.5-2 g/d divided in 3-4 doses x 7-10 days
Child > 8 years : 50 mg/kg/d divided in 3-4 doses x 7-10 days
or
erythromycin : same dosages as for tetracycline
or
cotrimoxazole
Adult   : 1600 mg of SMX/d divided in 2 doses x 7-10 days
Child   : 50 mg of SMX/kg/d divided in 2 doses x 7-10 days

If at the end of 3 courses of therapy the signs persist, consider tuberculosis (see "Tuberculosis", page 69).

Staphylococcal pneumonia

 Staphylococcal pneumonia often occurs in an infant that is otherwise unwell (malnutrition, skin sepsis…).

Clinical features

- Fever, pallor, fatigue.
- Signs similar to those of severe bronchiolitis, with vomiting, diarrhea, abdominal distension, often skin abscesses.
- Auscultation : asymmetrical chest signs + pleural effusion.
- Neutrophilia.
- Chest X-ray : bullæ, pleural effusion.

Treatment (hospital)

- Antibiotics, if available :
  cloxacillin (IV) : 100 mg/kg/d divided in 4 injections x 10 days
  and
  gentamicin (IM) : 3-6 mg/kg/d divided in 2 injections x 10 days
  Otherwise :
  chloramphenicol (IV) : 100 mg/kg/d divided in 3 injections x 10 days
- Hydration : oral or IV.
- If there is a significant effusion, a pleural tap may be necessary or, if severe, an intercostal catheter with underwater drain.

Prognosis

Danger of complications of suppurative pleurisy, pneumothorax and pyo-pneumothorax.

In a pediatric ward where staphylococcal pneumonia are expected to be managed, health workers should be trained to perform urgent pleural tap. Adequat equipment should always be available.

Bronchiolitis

 – Acute viral infection of the bronchioles occurring in infants under 10 months of age which can lead to fatal acute respiratory failure.
– Tends to occur in epidemics during the cold season.

Clinical features

– Onset often follows a cold.
– Low grade fever, cough, variable degree of respiratory distress with tachypnea, alar flare and chest indrawing (sternal and intercostal recession).
– Cyanosis if severe.
– Hyperinflated chest, hyper-resonant to percussion.
– Auscultation can be normal or reveal rhonchi (wheezes) and crepitations.

Treatment *(hospital)*

– Close monitoring : very important.
– Sitting position (propped up or held by mother).
– Keep well hydrated but avoid fluid overload.
– Humidified air.
– Bronchodilators : try *salbutamol* as a therapeutic test if available. The least dangerous is the spray (see "Asthma", see 67). Make two attempts at 15 minutes intervals, then wait. If there is improvement, continue ; if not, do not persist..
– *Corticosteroids* not effective.
– Antibiotics to prevent secondary bacterial infection :
cotrimoxazole (PO) : 40 mg of SMX/kg/day in 2 divided doses x 5 days
or
ampicillin (PO or IM) : 100 mg/kg/d divided in 3 doses x 5 days
– If cardiac decompensation (gallop rhythm, rate > 160) (see page 183) :
digoxin (IV) : 0.01 mg/kg stat every 6-8 hours for the first 24 hours thence same dose once daily as maintenance.
furosemide (IV) : 1 mg/kg
– Respiratory fatigue : if possible, intubation and manual ventilation.

Prognosis

– May have high mortality rate.
– Possibility of recurrence.

Asthma

 Paroxysmal reversible airways obstruction due to a combination of broncho-spasm, peribronchial edema and hypersecretion. Often allergic in origin.

2

Clinical features

– Wheeze (prolonged expiratory phase).
– Cough, dyspnea.
– Auscultation : expiratory rhonchi (wheezes) in both lung fields.
– 3 forms :
  • simple attack,
  • unstable asthma : repeated attacks,
  • status asthmaticus : prolonged, severe attack.

Treatment

Certain intestinal parasites during their invasive phase can cause allergic phenomena such as urticaria or asthma. Always think of this and treat in an endemic area : hookworm, strongyloides, ascaris, schistosomes, filaria.

SIMPLE ATTACK *(dispensary)*

– Half-sitting position, reassurance, hydration, oxygen if available.
– ***Aminophylline*** (PO) : 5 mg/kg every 6 hours as necessary (contra-indicated in children under 2 years).
– *Child < 2 years* : commence with ***salbutamol*** if available (the spray is the least dangerous), if not ***adrenaline*** (***epinephrine***) (see "alternative treatments", following page). Aminophylline should only be used as a last recours at this age.

SEVERE CASES = STATUS ASTHMATICUS *(hospital)*

– ***Aminophylline*** (IV) : 5 mg/kg diluted in 100 ml of 5% glucose, injected over 20 to 30 minutes. then 5 mg/kg over 6-8 hours depending on the clinical result.
– Never inject ***aminophylline*** undiluted (risk of convulsions and cardiac arrest).
– Combine with :
  • Infusions (alternative ***glucose*** and ***ringer lactate***)
  • ***salbutamol*** spray if avaiblable.
  • ***dexamethasone*** (IV) :
    Adult: 16-24 mg/d divided in 4-6 injections
    Child: 0.1-0.5 mg/kg/d divided in 4-6 injections
    Adjust the dosage to clinical state and decrease progressively.

– Antibiotics :
Adult   : ***peni V*** PO or ***PPF*** IM : 3-4 MIU/d x 5 days
Child < 5 years : ***chloramphenicol*** IV or PO : 100 mg/kg/d divided in 3-4 doses x 5 d
      or ***ampicillin*** IV or P : 100 mg/kg/d divided in 3-4 doses x 5 d

– After 2-3 hours aminophyllin infusion, when no improvement, return if possible to ***salbutamol*** or ***adrenaline***.

UNSTABLE CASES

– Attacks which stop and recur despite treatment.

– Institute the following
aminophylline (PO)
Adult and child : 8-12 mg/kg/d divided in 3 doses, reduce dose progressively
     over several days
Duration depends on clinical state ; decrease must be very gradual every 4-5 days.
Or better, but rarely available :
salbutamol (PO)
Adult : 12-16 mg/d divided in 3-4 doses x 5 days
Child : 0.2 mg/kg/d divided in 3-4 doses x 5 days, then decrease very gradualıy
   (every 4-5 days)

– In case of failure, consider short term, corticosteroid therapy. If used, it is essential
to exclude underlying pulmonary infection (if in doubt : ***peni V*** or ***cotrimoxazole***).
Give ***prednisone*** (or ***prednisolone***) per os
Adult : 30 mg/d in a single dose x 3-4 days
Childt : 1 mg/kg/d in a single dose x 3-4 days
Then decrease very gradually every 3-4 days depending on the clinical state.

ALTERNATIVE TREATMENTS

– ***salbutamol*** spray : a double puff if an attack occurs, without exceeding 3-4 doses per
day.

– ***salbutamol*** IV : difficult to control (tachycardia +++). Begin with 0.1 mg/10 kg in
100 ml 5 % glucose, over 20 minutes. Watch pulse, blood pressure.
Continue with 1 mg/hour (0.25-1.5 mg/h) for adult ; in child, 0.3-0.6 mg/10 kg/
hour. Change to oral treatment after 24 hours.
Reserve for refractory cases in children or status asthmaticus.

– ***epinephrine*** (***adrenaline***) SC : use 0.1 % (1 mg/ml) solution.
Adult : 0.5 ml SC, repeat if necessary 30 minutes later ; do not exceed 4 injections
   per day.
Child : 0.01 ml/kg SC without exceeding 0.5 ml/injection, repeat after
   30 minutes if still necessary ; do not exceed 4 injections per day ; exercise
   extreme caution (+++) in infants less than 1 year old.
Watch pulse, blood pressure (tachycardia +++).
Adrenaline can be utilised in case of simple attack.

Tuberculosis

☞ Disease of variable manifestations caused by Mycobacterium tuberculosis. It is important to understand the distinction between :

– Tuberculous infection : presence of M. *tuberculosis* in the organism, manifested by a positive skin test. Is very often asymptomatic.

– Tuberculous disease : affects about 10% of the infected population. Clinical disease can take very diverse forms :
  • meningitis,
  • pulmonary TB : the commonest form and the main source of transmission ("open" cases coughing up large numbers of AFB),
  • lymphadenitis,
  • osteo-articular, Pott's disease,
  • intestinal, renal, peritoneal, cutaneous

– Transmission and maintenance of endemicity depend upon :
  • the number and sources of infection : open pulmonary cases can be easily identified by 3 consecutive daily sputum examinations (direct smear for AFB) ;
  • living conditions : crowding, hygiene,
  • susceptibility of the population (e.g. malnutrition).

– Individuals with low immune defences (e.g. malnourished, infants, elderly, AIDS patients) are more susceptible to the very severe forms (TB meningitis, miliary TB).
  Note : not all cases of hemoptysis are necessarily TB. It is important not to forget other causes, especially if sputum smears are negative : paragonimiasis and meliodosis in Southeast Asia ; systemic mycoses ; histoplasmosis ; and bronchogenic carcinoma.

– An active pulmonary TB is considered as an opportunistic among AIDS or HIV infected patients, thus TB can be the initial step of AIDS.

Control of tuberculosis

ENVIRONMENT

Improvement of living conditions in a community lessens the risk of contagion (e.g. ventilation, light, no crowding...).

BCG AND CHEMOTHERAPY

– The *BCG* vaccination confers limited individual protection, and is mainly effective against infantile TB meningitis. It does not protect against most other forms of TB and does not confer herd immunity upon the population.

– The *chemotherapy* of TB is a complex issue. Certain fundamental rules must always be followed :

- Chemotherapy is only effective if rigorously organized and controlled. On an epidemiological level, a poorly organized program may be worse than no program at all. Poor treatment compliance leads to chronic, refractory cases and encourages the emergence of drug resistance.
- The success of a program depends less upon the intrinsic quality of the chosen treatment regimen than upon rigorous supervision and follow-up of patients during the entire duration of therapy.
- The program should be designed specifically for the local social, cultural and economic conditions.
- TB control is almost always co-ordinated at a national level. Foreign medical treams must adhere strictly to the national guidelines.

Practical organization

– The objective is to reduce transmission. The way to achieve this is to find and to treat sputum-positive cases.

– Clues to the identification of infectious patients are :
- cough of more than 3 weeks duration,
- hemoptysis, chest pain,
- weight loss,
- night sweats?

– Chest X-ray is not a particularly useful criterion for deciding upon treatment ; only sputum-positive and extrapulmonary cases should be commenced on therapy.

– The laboratory must be capable of carrying out direct smears for AFB, otherwise a control program cannot be envisaged. Active case detection is important, but only if a mechanism for effective treatment and follow-up exists.

– The main issue is to establish the mechanisms (infrastructure, trained personnel, transport, supplies) that will ensure good treatment compliance and follow-up, whatever the particular regimen. Without this, the program will fail. The availability of sophisticated drugs (such as rifampicin) is an issue of much lesser importance.

Three examples of treatment regimens

Low cost

Cost of full course < $US 20 ; 12 months duration.

– *isoniazid* (5mg/kg/d) + *thioacetazone* (2.5mg/kg/d) combination = *INH* + *TB1*
Adult   : tab 300 mg INH + tab 150 mg TB1
Child (< 6 years) : tab 100 mg INH + tab 50 mg TB1
each day by mouth for 12 months with an initial supplement of 2 months of *streptomycin* (IM) : 20 mg/kg

HIGH COST

Cost of full course > $US 175 ; 6 months duration.

– *isoniazid* : Adult : 5 mg/kg/d
   Child : 10 to 20 mg/kg/d
   + *rifampicin* : 10 mg/kg/d
   + *pyrazinamide* : 25 mg/kg/d for first 2 months only
   + *ethambutol* : 20 mg/kg/d for first 2 months only.

INTERMEDIATE COST

Cost of full course approx. $US 85 ; 8 months duration.

– First 2 months :
   isoniazid : 5 mg/kg/d
   + *rifampicin* : 10 mg/kg/d
   + *pyrazinamide* : 25 mg/kg/d
   + *streptomycin* (IM) : 20 mg/kg/d

– Next 6 months :
   isoniazid + *thioacetazone* : 5 mg/kg/d of INH.

Note

– Consult other documents on tuberculosis control programs, especially concerning case detection and short-course regimens (40).

– Hemoptysis is not always caused by tuberculosis. Other causes if AFB – : paragonimosis and melioïdosis in South East Asia ; deep mycosis : histoplasmosis ; bronchopulmonary cancer.

CHAPTER 3

Gastro-intestinal diseases

3

Stomatitis

☞ Inflammation of the oral mucosa, with or without infection, frequently found in infants.
If severe can contribute to malnutrition. Always treat carefully, and explain treatment to the mother.

Clinical features

– Sore mouth, dysphagia, anorexia, nausea, vomiting.

– Depending on etiology : red mucosa, aphthous or other ulcers, vesicles, white plaques.

Etiology and treatment

CANDIDA ALBICANS ("THRUSH") *(dispensary)*

– Common in infants.

– White plaques.

– Clean the mouth with a gauze swab soaked in *sodium bicarbonate*, then apply *gentian violet* with a cotton bud. Show the mother how to do this and have her repeat it 6 times a day.

– Often associated with gastro-intestinal candidosis. Treat all cases of oral thrush with :
nystatin (PO) : 100,000 to 200,000 IU/d divided in 3 doses x 5 to 10 days.
(Use the vaginal tablets if only these are available.)

– Educate the mother about oral hygiene.

– In severe forms, think of HIV infection.

HERPES SIMPLEX *(dispensary)*

Commoner in older children and adults. Infection causes pain and difficulty eating. Transmission is via microdroplets of saliva. Attacks are often preci-pitated by a febrile illness or stress.

– Oral toilet and apply *gentian violet*.

– Continued feeding and ensure good hydration.

– Treat any underlying illness (e.g. malaria, pneumonia).

– With a secondary infection (rare if good oral toilet) :
cotrimoxazole (PO)
Adult : 1,600 mg/d of SMX divided in 2 doses x 5 days
Child : 40 mg/kg/d of SMX divided in 2 doses x 5 days
or
chloramphenicol (PO) : 50 mg/kg/d divided in 3 doses x 5 days

SCURVY *(dispensary)*

Hemorrhagic stomatitis with bone and joint pains in the lower limbs (due to subperiosteal hemorrages). Caused by dietary vitamin C deficiency.

– Local treatment : oral toilet and *gentian violet.*

– Curative treatment
ascorbic acid (*vitamine C*)
Adult : 500-1000 mg/d divided in 3 doses during 2 to 3 weeks
Child : 100-300 mg/d divided in 3 doses during 2 to 3 weeks

– Preventive treatment
ascorbic acid (*vitamine C*)
Adult : 100 mg/d
Child : 30-50 mg/d
Nutritional education and supplementation with fresh fruit.

Other causes

– Vincent's angina (see page 51)

– Measles (Koplik's spot) (see pages 162-164)

– Diphtheria (see page 51)

– Scarlet fever (strawberry tongue) : a streptococcal infection.
Treatment :
PPF (or *procain penicillin*) : 100,000 IU/mg/d in a single injection x 5 days
then
penicillin V (PO) : same dose divided in 3 doses/d x 10 days

– Angular stomatitis of the lips : deficiencies in iron and various vitamins :
multivitamins
and/or
ferrous sulphate + folic acid (see pages 28-29)

Gastritis and Peptic Ulcer

☞ | Inflammatory or ulcerative lesions of the gastro-duodenal mucosæ.

3

Clinical features

– Epigastric burning pain, sometimes made worse and sometimes relieved by food (especially milk) but recurring about two hours after meals.
– Acid regurgitation, nausea.
– Abdomen soft and non-tender (unless perforation).
– Exclude parasitosis (strongyloides) : stool examination.

Treatment (dispensary)

– Diet : avoid spices, alcohol, tobacco, carbonated drinks. Encourage regular meals, dairy products.

– Antacids :
aluminium hydroxide (PO) : 300 to 500 mg in a single dose, taken 1 hour after each meal or during attacks of pain

– Reassure the patient : anxiety may be a causative factor. If needed :
diazepam (PO) : 15 mg/d divided in 3 doses for a <u>brief</u> period (5-10 days)

– If severe pain continues, exclude perforation : examine abdomen for peritonism, PR exam for rectal blood (melena on glove), keep under observation, surgical referral if necessary.
Give :
atropine (IM or SC) : 1 mg stat.

(hospital)

– If hemorrhage :
  • establish IV line,
  • give plasma volume expander (**Hæmacel**®...),
  • nasogastric tube : to observe if hemorrage continues,
  • transfuse if possible and refer to a surgical unit.

NB : *acetylsalicylic acid and other non-steroidal anti-inflammatories are contra-indicated in patients with a history of peptic ulcer.*

Acute diarrhoea

☞ Loose, frequent stools. Different cultures have different definitions, but as a guide, diarrhea means at least 3 loose or watery stools in a day.

Major complications :
– Dehydration : the principal reason for the mortality attributable to diarrhea
– Negative effect on nutritional status

Clinical assessment of the patient

HISTORY

– Duration of illness.

– Frequency and consistency of stools (blood, mucus).

– Frequency and duration of vomiting.

– Output, colour and quantity of urine.

– Fever or convulsions.

– Type and quantity of fluids and food ingested.

– Presence of blood or mucus in the stool.

– Presence of other cases in the household.

PHYSICAL EXAMINATION

– Temperature (rectal if possible).

– Respiration (acidosis : Kussmaul breathing).

– Weight :
  • as a baseline to monitor rehydration,
  • as an indicator of degree of dehydration.

– Nutritional status.

CLINICAL EVALUATION OF DEGREE OF DEHYDRATION

See table 4, page 79.

STOOL EXAMINATION

Direct smear, if available, to look for trophozoites of entamœba hystolitica or giardia lamblia.

Table 4 : *Clinical evaluation of dehydration*

SYMPTOMS AND SIGNS	MILD DEHYDRATION	MODERATE DEHYDRATION (2 signs present)	SEVERE DEHYDRATION (2 signs present)
General appearance – Young children	*Thirsty*, anxious, *alert*	*Thirsty, alert* or quiet but irritable when disturbed	*Drowsy*, floppy, cold, clammy, cyanosis, sometimes coma
– Older children and adults	Thirsty, alert	Thirsty, alert	Generally conscious, anxious, cold extremities, clammy, cyanosis, wrinkled skin of fingers, muscle cramps, dizzy if standing
Pulse	Normal	Rapid	Rapid, thready, sometimes absent
Respiration	Normal	Deep, sometimes rapid	Deep and rapid
Anterior fontanelle (6 to 18 months)	Normal	*Depressed*	*Severely depressed*
Systolic BP	Normal	Normal	Low, sometimes unmeasurable
Skin elasticity	*Normal : fold of pinched skin disappears at once*	*Decreased*	*Fold disappears very slowly* (> 2 seconds)
Eyes	Normal	*Sunken*	*Severely sunken*
Tears	Present	Absent	Absent
Mucous membranes (test mouth with a clean finger)	Moist	Dry	Very dry
Urine output	Normal	*Reduced, urine dark*	*Anuria, empty bladder*
% of body weight lost	1 – 5 %	6 – 9 %	10 % and more
Estimated fluid deficit	10 – 50 ml/kg	60 – 90 ml/kg	100 ml/kg

3

Etiology

Table 5

ETIOLOGY		SYMPTOMS AND SIGNS	CAUSATIVE AGENTS	TREATMENT
Entero-invasive	Bacteria	Dysentery, blood and mucus in stools, cramps, tenesmus, fever	Shigella Salmonella Escherichia Coli (EIEC strains)	*Cotrimoxazole* *Ampicillin* *Chloramphenicol* *Tetracycline*
			Campylobacter jejuni	*Erythromycin* *Tetracycline*
			Yersinia Enterolitica	*Chloramphenicol* *Tetracycline* *Cotrimoxazole* *Gentamicin*
	Parasites	As above, but usually no fever (except with amœbic liver abscess)	Entamœba hystolitica Giardia lamblia	*Metronidazole*
			Balantidium Coli	*Metronidazole* *Tetracycline*
Enterotoxix bacteria		Cholera-like illness : profuse watery diarrhoea (rice water, stools), often vomiting	Vibrio choleræ	*Tetracycline* *Erythromycin* *Furazolidone*
			Other vibrios	As above
			Enterotoxic E. coli (ETEC strains)	*Cotrimoxazole* *Ampicillin* *Chloramphenicol*
			Clostridium perfringens Botulinum Staphylococcus	No treatment (toxins preformed in foodstuffs)
			Aeromonas Céreus bacilli	
Viral (60 % of cases)		Liquid diarrhoea, no mucus, sometimes fever. Commonest in infants and young children	Rotavirus, Entero-virus, Adenovirus, Astrovirus, Corona-virus	Antibiotic treatment no recommended
Fungal		Diarrhoea often asso-ciated with oral thrush. Fungi evident on stools microscopy	Candida Albicans	*Nystatin*

Treatment

Basic principles :

– Prevent dehydration.

– Replace fluid if dehydration already exists.

– Maintain nutrition.

PREVENTION OF DEHYDRATION

Cases of diarrhea with no signs of dehydration :

– Advise increasing fluid intake (water, soup, juices, rice water).

– Encourage the use of home-made sugar/salt solutions.

– Continue breast feeding and normal diet.

– Warn mother to bring child back if :
  • signs of dehydration appear (explain),
  • diarrhea persists.

FLUID REPLACEMENT

– Two tasks :
  • Rehydration : correct the deficit in water and electrolytes.
  • Maintenance : replace continuing losses (diarrhea and vomiting).

– Two methods of fluid replacement :
  • *ORS* : for mild to moderate dehydration, give by mouth or by nasogastric tube if child unable or unwilling to drink.
  • *Ringer's lactate* : for severe dehydration or if there is intractable vomiting.

– Quantities of fluid are calculated according to the condition of the patient (see tables 6 and 7, pages 82 and 83). As a general rule, for severe dehydration 200 ml/kg/day should be given with the first half during the first 4 hours. For moderate dehydration, give 100 ml/kg/day with first half given during first 4 hours.

– Mild cases can be treated as outpatients, after the mother has been shown how to use *ORS*. Moderate and severe cases require supervision as to the evolution of the diarrhea and progress of rehydration.

– If it is impossible to place an IV line in a severely dehydrated child, fluids are sometimes given intraperitoneally or subcutaneously. However these techniques should not be encouraged, as they are less safe and no more effective than giving ORS by nasogastric tube.

Note : *solution of salt-sugar* : 2 pinches of salt (3 g), 4 tablespoons of sugar, or 8 pieces (40 g), dissolved in 1 liter of boiled water, cooled and with added fruit juice.

Table 6 : *Rehydration protocol*

– The volumes indicated are guides only.

– Before using this table, consider all of the following :

- *Rehydration must be evaluated in terms of clinical signs, not in terms of volume of fluids given.*
- *If necessary, the volumes given below can be increased or else the initial high rate of administration can be maintained until there is clinical improvement.*
- Periorbital edema is a sign of fluid overload in infants.
- Maintenance therapy (table 7) should begin *as soon as* signs of dehydration have resolved, but *not before.*

DEGREE OF DEHYDRATION	TYPE OF LIQUID	VOLUME TO GIVE
Mild	*ORS*	As needed (do not force) Theorically, 50 ml/kg in 4 hours
Moderate	*ORS*	100 ml/kg/d of which half (50 ml/kg) in first 4 hours and rest (50 ml/kg) in following 20 hours[a]
	Ringer or *Hartman*[b]	100 ml/kg/d of which half (50 ml/kg) in first 4 hours and rest (50 ml/kg) in following 20 hours
Severe	*Ringer* or *Hartman*[b]	200 ml/kg/d of which half (100 ml/kg) in first 4 hours and rest (100 ml/kg) in following 20 hours

[a] Initially, adults can usually ingest up to 750 mg o ORS/hour, and children about 300 ml/hour.

[b] If ringer's lactate (Hartman's solution) is not available, use :
- Half strength Darrow's solution
- normal saline with sodium bicarbonate and potassium chloride added
- normal saline diluted to half strength with 5 % glucose (dextrose)

None of these solutions is as effective as ringer's lactate.

W.H.O. (36)

Table 7 : *Maintenance therapy*

Notes :

− fluids to be given after correction of dehydration ;

− adapt re-hydration treatment to the clinical status of the patient ;

− to avoid hypernatremia alternate *ORS* and water.

SEVERITY OF DIARRHOEA	FLUID	ADMINISTRATION	QUANTITY
Mild diarrhoea (no more than 1 stool every 2 hours, or less than 5 ml/kg of stools per hour)	*ORS*	Orally : at home	Infants and children under 5 years[a] : 100 ml/kg/day until diarrhoea ceases Older children and adults : as much as desired[b]
Severe diarrhoea (more than 1 stool every 2 hours, or more than 5 ml/kg of stools per hour)	*ORS*	Orally : at the health care facility	Replace the same volume that is lost through continuing diarrhoea. If stool volumes cannot be measured, give as for moderate diarrhoea.
Severe diarrhoea with *reappearance* of signs of *dehydration*	Treat as for severe dehydration (see table 6)		

[a] As weel as ORS give the breast on demand. Other liquids such as plain water can also be given. ORS should consitute about two thirds of the fluid intake until diarrhoea ceases.

[b] Thirst is the best guide for maintenance fluid therapy in older children and adults. They should drink as much ORS (and other liquids) as they desire.

W.H.O. (36)

MAINTAIN NUTRITION

It has been shown that there is no physiological reason for discontinuing food during bouts of diarrhea and that continued nutrition is beneficial to both adults and children. Continued feeding should be encouraged.

Table 8 : *Infant feeding*

AGE	BREAST FEEDING	OTHER FOODS
0 – 3 months	Begin breast feeding immediately after delivery Feeding on demand	Nil (unless mother cannot breast feed)
4 – 6 months	Continue	Add at least two other food* .... Twice a day
6 – 12 months	Continue	Add other foods* as well .... Four times a day
After 1 year	Continue till about 2 years of age	All foods Four to six times a day

* These "weaning foods" (a poor term, as breast feeding must continue) should include : energy-rich porridges (staple carbohydrate with oils and sugar added if possible), vegetables, fruit and animal protein.

W.H.O. (36)

MEDICINES

– Remember that 50-60 % of acute gastro-enteritis is viral (see table 5, page 80).
– Certain antibiotics are used to treat specific intestinal infections.

Table 9 : *Antibiotics used in the treatment of diarrhoea*

ETIOLOGY	FIRST CHOICE	ALTERNATIVES
Cholera	*Tetracycline* per os Adult : 1.5-2 g/d divided in 3 doses x 2-3 days Child : 50 mg/kg/d divided in 3 doses x 2-3 days or *Doxycycline* per os Adult : 300 mg single dose	*Furazolidone* or *Nitrofurantoin* per os Adult : 400 mg/d divided in 3 doses x 3 days Child : 5 mg/kg/d divided in 3 doses x 3 days or *Cotrimoxazole* per os Adult : 1,600 mg of SMX/d divided in 2 doses x 3 days Child : 50 mg of SMX/kg/d divided in 2 doses x 3 days
Shigella dysentery	*Cotrimoxazole* per os Adult : 1,600 mg ofSMX/d divided in 2 doses x 5 days Child : 50 mg of SMX/kg/d divided in 2 doses x 5 days	*Nalidixic acid* per os Adult : 3 g/d divided in 3 doses x 5 days Child : 60 mg/kg/d divided in 3-4 doses x 5 days or *Ampicillin* per os Adult : 3-4 g/d divided in 3-4 doses x 5 days Child : 100 mg/kg/d divided in 3-4 doses x 5 days
Intestinal amœbiasis (acute amœbic dysentery)	*Metronidazole* per os Adult : 1.5-2 g/d divided in 3 doses x 5 days Child : 30-50 mg/kg/d divided in 3 doses x 5 days (10 days for severe amœbiasis)	
Giardiasis	*Metronidazole* per os Adult : 750 mg/d divided in 3 doses x 5 days Child : 15 mg/kg/d divided in 3 doses x 5 days	

W.H.O. (36)

– **Other anti-diarrhoea indications (e.g. absorbents) are contraindicated in children.**
– Always treat the fever and consider other causes for the diarrhoea (e.g. malaria, otitis, pneumonia).

Prevention of diarrhea

HEALTH EDUCATION

Directed at mothers in dispensaries, MCH clinics and feeding centers, at the time ORS is prescribed.

Take-home messages :
1) Breastfeeding :
   - on its own up to age 4 months
   - continue up to age 2 years
2) **Solid** foods ("weaning foods" is a very poor term) : introduce these from about age 4 months
3) Food preparation
4) Drinking water
5) Hygiene

SANITATION

– Provision of safe drinking water in sufficient quantities
– Disposal of feces

MASS CHEMOPROPHYLAXIS

– This is only ever considered in cholera epidemics. It is of doubtful efficacy in controlling an outbreak and can only be justified in a sequestered populations : a ship, a medium size where the attack rate is high (more than 2 %) and where it is possible to administer an effective prophylactic dose under supervision to the whole group concerned.
– In endemic situation, it can be given to close family contacts.
– **Doxycycline** should be choosen.

Note

Composition of ORS sachets
(to be dissolved in 1 litre of clean water (do not tell mothers to boil the water as this is very expensive in terms of time and fuel, and also unnecessary).

Ingredients	*Grammes*
Sodium chloride	3,5
Sodium bicarbonate or	2,9
Trisodium citrate	2,5
Potassium chloride	1,5
Glucose	20,0

CHAPTER 4

Skin conditions

4

Dermatology

☞ Infections and infestations are by far the most frequent forms of skin pathology in tropical countries. As well as treating affected individuals, it is important to consider these conditions as indicators of the general standard of hygiene and sanitation and to define appropriate public health interventions (provision of water that is adequate in quality and quantity, health education, soap…).

Clinical assessment of the patient

The physical examination :

– Describe the *basic lesions* :
  • macules
  • papules
  • vesicles
  • bullæ
  • abscess
  • pustules
  • squames
  • weeping lesions
  • crusts…

– Look for pruritis.

– Look for *regional or systemic manifestations* : lymphangitis, adenopathy, fever, septicemia, metastatic infection…

– Look for a cause : mosquito bite, jewelry, allergy, scabies, lice, otitis media.

– Consider the nutritional status and the general health of the family, particularly for infectious dermatosis.

Patients with dermatological conditions often present late. At this stage, initial and specific signs are often replaced by infection. In these cases, treating the overlying infection is not enough. Patients should be re-examined after the treatment of infection.

4

Impetigo and other purulent dermatoses

☞ | Highly contagious skin infection (streptococcal or staphylococcal affecting mainly children of school age).

Clinical features

- Initially lesions located around orifices.
- Multiple crusty lesions, sometimes associated with pustules (one to several). Lesions are extended by scratching
- Acute impetigo produces bullous lesions.
- Streptococcal lesions are superficial, staphylococcal lesions are deep.

Treatment (dispensary)

- Cut fingernails, instruct mother to wash child daily with soap.
- Clean lesions with a disinfectant (**chloramine** or **chlorhexidine-cetrimide** solution ; preparation : see table 25, page 221). Remove crusts, incise any abscesses.
- Apply **gentian violet** solution twice daily.
- On the scalp look for head lice or ringworm (tinea capitis). If present, shave the head and treat as page 95.
- Explain treatment to the mother and treat other members of the family as necessary.
- Do not give antibiotics unless there are signs of regional or systemic spread. If so :
  penicillin V (PO)
  Adult : 2.4 MIU/d divided in 3 doses x 5 days
  Child : 100,000 mg/kg/d divided in 3 doses x 5 days
  If no improvement or extensive abscesses, staphylococcal infection is likely. If available give :
  erythromycin (PO) : 50 mg/kg/d divided in 3 doses x 5 days
  or **cloxacillin** (PO) : 100 mg/mg/d divided in 3 doses x 5-7 days
- Carbuncles on the face. There is a danger of intracerebral metastasis, so treat vigorously for 5-7 days.
  If available :
  cloxacillin (IV or PO) : 100 mg/kg/d divided in 4 injections x 7 days
  or **chloramphenicol** (IV) : 75 mg/kg/d divided in 4 injections x 7 days
  or
  ampicillin (IV) : 100 mg/kg/d divided in 4 injections x 7 days
  + gentamicin (IM) : 3 mg/kg/d divided in 2 or 3 injections x 7 days

Herpes simplex, Herpes zoster

Herpes simplex

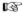 Relapsing vesicular eruption due to Herpes simplex virus affecting the mucus membranes and skin. Facial infections may be serious if they involve the eye.

Treatment *(dispensary)*

– Clean the lesions with an antiseptic such as ***chlorhexidine-cetrimide*** solution (dilution : see table 25, page 221).
– If affecting buccal mucosa then treat as for stomatitis.
– If affecting the face encourage ocular hygiene (see pages 105-106).
– If generalized bacterial super infection, treat as for staphylococcal impetigo (see previous page).

Herpes zoster

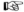 Acute dermatosis due to resurgence of the varicella-zoster virus, which also causes chickenpox. Preceded by severe neuralgic pain, the eruption is vesicular on an erythematous base and is almost invariably unilateral, occupying the dermatome of a peripheral nerve.

Treatment *(dispensary)*

As above, plus analgesia (see pages 22-23).

Scabies

 Contagious skin infestation caused by a mite, Sarcoptes scabiei. Its occurrence is closely related to a lack of water and poor hygiene.

Clinical picture

- Nocturnal itching, scratch marks, burrows between the fingers (made visible by applying ink, then washing it off), and papules.
- Secondary infection (from scratching) resembles impetigo.
- Whole family is often infested.
- Often localised to : genital region, axillæ, chest, breasts, hands and thighs.

Treatment (dispensary)

- Wash the whole body with a mild soap and dry, then apply 25 % *benzyl benzoate emulsion* (*BBE*) to the whole body except head and neck. Use a broad paint brush if available. Allow to dry, then put on the same clothes.
- Repeat for 3 days.
- If a secondary bacterial infection occurs, treat as for impetigo (see page 90) for 4 to 5 days. Only apply *benzyl benzoate emulsion* once all lesions are closed (is very irritant).
- Treat the whole family. After the treatment, boil and air all clothes and bedding.
- Warn patients that itching may persist for several weeks. This represents an allergic reaction to the dead mites, not treatment failure.

Leg ulcer

☞ | Erosive lesion of the skin, usually occurring on the lower leg caused by :
– vascular (venous and / or arterial) insufficiency,
– bacterial or parasitic infection,
– underlying metabolic disorders.
Phadegenic ulcers have no apparent cause, they extend and become chronic.

Treatment (dispensary)

– Clean with *chlorhexidine-cetrimide* or *chloramin* solutions (dilution : see table 25, page 221).

– Excise necrotic edges.

– Daily dressing.

– Rest with leg elevated.

– Give oral antibiotics if local treatment fails :
penicillin V (PO) :
Adult : 2.4 MIU / d divided in 3 doses x 5 days
Child : 100,000 IU / kg / d divided in 3 doses x 5 days
If no improvement, give :
erythromicin (PO) : 50 mg / kg / d divided in 3 doses x 7 days

– Skin graft (see pages 230-231) if ulcer is large. Only graft after local treatment has rendered it clean and flat with red granulation tissue in the base.

Note

– Think of Guinea worm in endemic zones.

– Give tetanus toxoid (see pages 147-148).

4

Fungal infection

Infant's thrush

Clinical features

Erythema of the buttocks and perineum, sometimes "weeping". Caused by infection with Candida albicans.

Treatment (*dispensary*)

– Clean with usual soap or an antiseptic (***chloramine*** or ***chlorhexidine-cetrimide*** ; preparation : see table 25, page 221).

– Apply ***gentian violet*** solution twice daily.

– Avoid damp clothing (leave buttocks bare).

– Intestinal thrush often co-exists :
Nystatin (PO) : 4-600,000 IU/d divided in 3 doses x 10 days (vaginal tabs might be used for this purpose)

Dermatoses

 Highly contagious fungal infections. Prevalence is associated with the level of personal hygiene.

Clinical features

BODY

There are several different forms :

– "Ringworm"

– Pityriasis versicolor with depigmented patches.

– Erythematous lesions in the skin folds (e.g. axillæ and groin).

HEAD

Associated with loss of hair. Highly contagious in families.

Treatment

BODY *(dispensary)*

– Wash, dry and then apply *whitfield's ointment* twice a day.

– Use *griseofulvin* only in extensive cases (see below).

HEAD *(dispensary)*

– Cut hair and then shave the head.

– Wash, dry and then apply *gentian violet* twice a day for several weeks.

– If treatment fails use :
griseofulvin (PO)
Adult : 500 mg to 1 g/d divided in 3 doses
Child : 10 mg/kg/d divided in 3 doses
Treat for 10 days (sometimes treatment has to be continued for 1 month).

– Examine all the family.

– A short course of griseofulvin may be effective for adults :
griseofulvin : 1.5 g taken at the same time as a greasy meal.
However, there is a risk of digestive problems and vertigo.

4

Anthrax

 A bacterial zoonosis of herbivorous mammals that is transmitted to humans by skin contact with carcasses or animal products, and rarely by ingestion of undercooked infected meat.

Clinical features

– Pustule that develops into a black eschar surrounded by vesicles and an inflamed area, with regional adenopathy. **Painless.**
– May cause fatal septicemia.
– Intestinal and pulmonary forms exist.

Treatment *(hospital)*

penicillin : **PPF** (or **procain penicilline**) IM
Adult : 4 MU/d in a single injection x 5 days
Child : 100,000 U/kg/d in a single injection x 5 days

or
penicillin V
Adult : 4 MU/d divided in 3 doses x 7 days
Child : 100,000 U/kg/d divided in 3 doses x 7 days

or
chloramphenicol per os
Adult : 1.5-2 g/d divided in 3 doses x 7 days
Child : 75 mg/kg/d divided in 3 doses x 7 days

or
tetracycline per os
Adult   : 1.5-2 g/d divided in 3-4 doses x 7 days
Child > 8 years : 50 mg/kg/d divided in 3-4 doses x 7 days

Prevention

Look for the source of contamination and take measures to prevent further transmission.

Other skin conditions

Eczema (dermatitis)

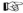 – Erythema with crusting, scaling, itching, and desquamation.
– Look for a cause (e.g. irritants, allergic, fungal, family history).

Treatment *(dispensary)*

4

– Apply *gentian violet* solution. If infected, treat as for impetigo.

– If chronic, consider an eczematized scabies infestation and treat appro-priately.

Urticaria

 – Rapidly developing itchy papules.
– Look for a cause (e.g. insect bites, drug allergy, invasive stage of a parasitic infection of ascaris, hookworm, strongyloides, schisto-somiasis or loa-loa).

Treatment *(dispensary)*

– Intense itching :
promethazine (PO) : 75 mg/d divided in 3 doses x 5 days
or
chlorphenamine (PO) : 12 mg/d divided in 3 doses

– Angiedema (laryngeal or pharyngeal involvement).
dexamethasone (IV) : 4 mg (repeat if necessary)

– If anaphylactic shock, see "Shock", page 33.

Kwashiorkor

- Multiple lesions : desquamation,, bullas...
- To prevent secondary infection, clean lesions with either *chloramine* or *chlorhexidine-cetrimide* solution and apply *gentian violet* (see table 25, page 221).

Pellagra

Dermatosis affecting sun-exposed skin due to a dietary deficiency in niacin and/or tryptophane. Commonest in populations whose staple carbohydrate is maize.

Clinical features

- Classically, "three D's" : dermatitis, diarrhea and dementia.
- The dermatitis is painful, more marked in sun-exposed areas of forehead, neck, forearms and legs... symmetrical.
- Diarrhoea and neurological symptoms indicating serious illness.

Treatment (dispensary)

- Use :
  nicotamide (*vitamin PP*)
  Adult : 300 mg/d
  Child : 300 mg/d
  until healing is complete and in conjunction with a rich protein diet.
- If unavailable, use :
  multivitamins (PO)
  Adult : 6 caps/d divided in 3 doses x 15 days
  Child : 3 caps/d divided in 3 doses x 15 days
- Provide nutritional education (e.g. diversify staples, advise vegetables such as beans and lentils).

Note

Leprosy may in some instances resemble a chronic dermatosis such as eczema or pityriasis versicolor. Whenever there is the slightest doubt, perform a full examination of the peripheral nerves and take specimens for microscopy.

Endemic syphilis, Yaws & Pinta

☞ Non-venereal treponematoses, affecting bone, skin or mucosa and spread by direct contact. Their occurrence is associated with over crowding and poor hygiene.

Table 10 : *The treponematoses*

	VENERAL SYPHILIS	BEJEL	YAWS	PINTA
– *Causative agent*	T. Pallidum (veneral)	T. Pallidum (endemic)	T. Pertenue	T. Carateum
– *Mode of transmission*	Veneral sometimes	Contact	Contact (flies)	Contact (black flies)
– *Age*	Adult	Child	Child	All ages
– *Distribution*	Cosmopolitan	Deserts Plains	Tropical forest	Latin America
– *Primary infection*	Genital chancre	0	Non genital chancre	"Pseudomy-cotic" lesion
– *Secondary infection* *skin*	Rash lesions	Lesions	Wart-like lesion changes Hyperkeratosis	Pigmentary
mucus membranes	Mucous patches	Mucous patches	Gangosa	0
bone	Osteitis	Osteitis +	Osteitis ++	0
– *Tertiary infection* *skin*	+	+	+	0
gumma	+	+	+ ⎤ gangosa	0
osteitis	+	+	+ ⎟	0
cardio-vascular	+	+	⎦ 0	0
CNS	+	+	0	0
– *Congenital transmission*	+	0	0	0

Adapted from M. Gentilini (10)

4

Treatment *(dispensary)*

– **benzathine penicillin** (IM)
Adult : 1.2 MIU in a single injection
Child : 600,000 IU in a single injection

– Note that syphilis (both primary and secondary) must be treated with double this dose of
benzathine penicillin : 2.4 MIU IM stat.

– If allergic to penicillin :
tetracycline or **erythromycin** (PO) : 2 g/d or 50 mg/kg/d divided in 3 doses x 5 days (14 days for syphilis)

Prophylaxis

– For all household contacts :
benzathine penicillin (IM)
Adult : 600,000 IU in a single injection
Child : 300,000 IU in a single injection

Leprosy

 A chronic infectious disease caused by the Hansen bacillus (Mycobacterium lepræ) and affecting the skin, mucosæ and peripheral nerves. Humans are the only significant reservoir of infection.

Clinical features

COMPLETE CLINICAL EXAMINATION

– Patient must be undressed.
– The entire skin surface must be examined.
– Note the appearance of any lesions.
– Test the sensation (fine touch and pin-prick) of the lesions.
– Palpate the main peripheral nerves to detect any hypertrophy.
– Examine peripheral nervous function : motor, sensory and proprioception.
– Examine the nasal mucosa to detect any chronic rhinitis.

MICROBIOLOGICAL EXAMINATION

Ziehl-Nielsen stain
– Scraped incision method to obtain tissue juice but no blood. Pinch a fold of skin with a Kocher forceps so as to make it bloodless, incise and scrape the scalpel blade along the inside of the incision.
  • one specimen from the edge of a lesion.
  • one from the earlobe.
– Also take a nasal swab.

CLASSIFICATION (RIDLEY-JOPLING SYSTEM)

FEW BACILLI			MANY BACILLI	
Tuberculoid	Borderline Tuberculoid	Borderline	Borderline Lepromatous	Lepromatous
T.T.	B.T.	B.B.	B.L.	L.L.

Principles of management

The increasing frequency of strains of M. leprae resistant to dapsone poses a serious threat to leprosy control programs. The strategy of multiple drug therapy must be instituted in order to combat this problem.

It is patients with multibacillary forms of leprosy (BL and LL) who are most exposed to the risk of drug resistance and who are also most infectious to their household contacts.

The treatment of lepromatous leprosy has three objectives :
1. to reduce transmission
2. to cure the patient
3. **to prevent the emergence of resistant strains of M. leprae**

Patients with tuberculoid leprosy are less infectious but are more likely to suffer paralysis of peripheral nerves. The main objective of their treatment is to preserve function.

Patients under therapy are exposed to the risk of developing **severe reactions**. For this reason, as well as to ensure compliance, **supervision is necessary. The program must be well planned, organized and adequately staffed.**

Treatment

"Partially supervised" regimens work best. Daily doses of dapsone can be taken at home by the patient, but monthly doses of rifampicin should be administered by a health worker. The worker must ensure that the patient swallows the medication

LEPROMATOUS LEPROSY *(dispensary)*

rifampicin   (PO) : 600 mg once per month, supervised
dapsone   (PO) : 100 mg daily, at home
clofazimine (PO) : 300 mg once per month, supervised
                                   and 50 mg daily, at home

Duration of therapy : 2 years or more, depending upon progress

TUBERCULOID LEPROSY *(dispensary - hospital)*

rifampicin   (PO) : 600 mg once per month, during 6 months
dapsone   (PO) : 100 mg daily during 6 months (1-2 mg/kg/day)

– *rifampicin* must always be taken under supervision.

– *dapsone* may be taken at home. If treatment is interrupted, a full 6 months regimen should be completed after the medication has been discontinued.

REACTIONS

– Either reversal reactions (upgrading : shift towards TT end of spectrum) or erythema nodosum leprosum (ENL).

– Treat with *clofazimine* (PO) : 100 to 300 mg/d

– If severe, use corticosteroids :
   prednisone (or *prednisolone*) PO : 80 mg D1 ; 75 mg D2 ; 70 mg D3 ; 65 mg D4 ; 60 mg D5... then decrease 5 mg every day.

CHAPTER 5

Eye conditions

5

Conjunctivitis

☞
- Acute inflammation of the conjunctivæ which may be infectious (viral or bacterial), allergic or irritative.
- Infectious conjunctivitis is often endemic and may become epidemic in conditions of poor hygiene. Secondary infection may lead to keratitis and subsequent blindness.
- Viral conjunctivitis is often preceded by a cold.

Clinical features

- "Red eye" (injected conjunctivæ), either unilateral or bilateral. May be purulent discharge. Visual acuity intact.

- Pain and photophobia are signs of corneal involvement. Look for pericorneal injection and examine after fluoroscein staining if available. Examine carefully to exclude foreign body (corneal or conjunctival).

- Chronic pruritis is usually the allergic form.

5

Treatment

(dispensary)

- **Usual picture**

  • Wash a several times a day to remove any discharge. Use cooled boiled water or normal saline.
  • Then, apply :
    tetracycline eye ointment 1 % : 4 times/day x 5 days
    or *sulphacetamide* 10 % .
  • Always look for foreign bodies (sub-conjuctival or corneal) and remove.
  • Never use topical steroids.

(hospital)

- **Ophthalmia neonatorum (gonococcal)**

  It is bilateral and appears immediately after birth. If only after 3 days, it is likely to be chlamydia.

  • Prevention

    Formerly, a 1% solution of *silver nitrate* was used for all neonates. This product is effective but may be dangerous if poorly prepared or stored ; evaporation in hot climates may greatly increase the solution's concentration and thus toxicity. The current WHO recommendation is to use :
    tetracycline 1% eye ointment : apply in each eye at birth.

• Treatment

Clean with *normal saline* or *ringer's lactate* at least 4 times/day (danger of sticking).
+ *tetracycline* 1% eye ointment applied 2 hourly initially.
+ *penicillin G* (IM) : 100,000 IU/kg divided in 3-4 injections x 7 days.
Treat the mother (see page 194).

– *Allergic conjunctivitis*

Treat as for simple conjunctivitis.
+ *promethazine* (PO) : 75 mg/d divided in 3 doses
or *chlorphenamine* (PO) : 12 mg/d divided in 3 doses

– *Keratoconjunctivitis* (corneal ulcers)

Same treament as for simple conjunctivitis : *tetracyclin* ointment. Never use ointments or drops containing corticosteroids.
Give *vitamin A* in therapeutic doses (see page 108) and cover with an eye pad to relieve pain and photophobia. Oral analgesia as needed.
Consult ophthalmologist whenever one is available.
If too painful, *adrenaline* (*epinephrine*) can be given (dilution of 1 mg ampoule in 10 ml normal saline or ringer's lactate) : apply several drops 4 times/day.

– *Prophylaxis against the ocular complications of systemic conditions* (e.g. measles and other febrile illnesses) :

vitamin A in prophylactic doses (see page 108).
Prophylactic eye toilet with 0.9 % *ringer's lactate* solution.

Trachoma

☞
— Keratoconjunctivitis **due to Chlamydia trachomatis**. It is the world's major cause of blindness.
— **Endemic and contagious**, its occurrence is associated with poor hygiene, lack of water and over crowding.

Clinical features

Trachoma evolves through **four stages**. Early forms (stages I and II) can be completely cured with appropriate therapy. Patients in endemic areas should be examined by everting the upper eyelid (have the patient look down and draw the eyelashes up while "tripping" the tarsal plate over a matchstick).
Follicles are the basic lesions ; there are whitish granulations on an inflammatory base. Staging is discussed below.

Treatment

Treatment is always local. WHO does not recommend systemic antibiotics, though these were formerly used. The regimen alters according to the staging of the illness.

STAGE I *(dispensary)*
— Bilateral follicular conjunctivitis, first present in the upper palpebral conjunctiva (thus the need always to evert the upper lid).
— *tetracycline* 1% eye ointment 3 times / day x 4-6 weeks.

STAGE II *(dispensary)*
— Frank trachoma : as in stage I, plus vascular pannus across cornea.
— Same treatment as above, for 2 to 3 months.

STAGE III *(dispensary)*
— Scarring and infiltration of the palpebral and bulbar conjunctivæ and of the cornea. Complete cure is no longer possible.
— Local disinfection and *tetracycline* ointment.

STAGE IV *(dispensary)*
— Scarring and contractures invert the edge of the lids producing an entropion.
— Irritation by eyelashes (trichiasis) causes more severe ulceration and scarring of the cornea. Blindness results.
— Only surgical treatment is effective in correcting the entropion. Surgery should be offered even if the patient is already blind, so as to reduce continuing irritation and pain.
— If infection remains active, administer *tetracycline* ointment.

Prevention

— Adequate quantities of soap and water
— Personal hygiene (hand washing, eye toilet)
— Health education

5

Vitamin A deficiency

☞ Nutritional deficiency of vitamin A principally affecting infants and young children. Clinical manifestations are often precipitated by an acute febrile illness (measles, diarrhea etc) and signs may evolve very quickly (in hours).

Clinical features

STAGE I

Night blindness

Difficult to observe in infants and young children, but at nightfall they may stop playing or become fearful.

STAGE II

Xerophthalmia

Dryness (xerosis) affecting first the conjunctivæ then the cornea.
Bitot's spots : foamy white patches on bulbar conjunctiva.

STAGE III

Keratomalacia

Corneal opacities, quickly leading to blindness.

Treatment (dispensary)

Only stages I and II are completely reversible.

Give *vitamin A* at all stages of active xerophtalmia. Also give vitamin A to all children with measles. Corneal changes require urgent treatment.
– 100,000 IU stat PO for infants < 1 year on day 1, day 2 and day 8.
– 200,000 IU stat PO for older children and adults on day 1, day 2 and day 8.

Prevention

– Vitamin A

- Mother : 200,000 IU at the time of delivery or in the two months which follow. Fertile women must not receive more than 10,000 IU/d, except in the two months following a delivery.

- Children from 6 to 11 months of age : 100,000 IU by mouth every 3 to 6 months.

- Children from 1 to 5 years of age : 200,000 IU by mouth every 3 to 6 months.

– Nutritional education : instruct mothers on locally available foods that are rich in vitamin A (e.g. yellow fruits, vegetables - especially papaya and carrots - red palm oil, green leafy vegetables, liver, eggs...).

Note : doses of vitamin A given should be marked on the health card. It is toxic so do not exceed the recommended dose.

5

Pterygium

☞ – Whitish triangular membrane on the nasal aspect of the bulbar conjunctiva, progressing slowly towards the cornea.
– Associated with dry climates, dust and wind. Does not regress spontaneously.

Treatment (dispensary)

– *Uncomplicated pterygium*
Symptomless, not encroaching across the pupil. No treatment.

– *Progressive pterygium*
Vascular, encroaching across the pupil, causing discomfort, lacrimation and sometimes secondary infection :

• Disinfection : wash eye with *normal saline*, apply *tetracycline* ointment.

• Surgical excision : if skills and facilities are available locally.

Cataract

☞ Bilateral opacities of the lens that cause a progressive loss of visual acuity.

Cataract is common in tropical regions and occurs at a younger age than in Western countries. It is possibly associated with repeated episodes of dehydration.

Apart from surgery there is no treatment.

5

Onchocerciasis

See pages 119-121.

CHAPTER 6

Parasitic diseases

6

Schistosomiasis *(blood flukes)*

PARASITE	MODE OF TRANSMISSION	SIGNS	TREATMENT	PREVENTION
S. Hematobium (Tropical and North Africa, Middle East)	Transcutaneous during contact with water conta- minated with cercariae BULINUS SPP	Dysuria, haematuria Late : hydronephrosis Eggs in urine	**Metrifonate** per os Adult : 600 mg Child : 10 mg/kg divided en 2 doses at 2 weekly intervals Alternative : **praziquantel** see S. Intercalatum	Avoid swimming Health education Vector control Mass chemotherapy
S. Mansoni (Tropical Africa, Latin America)	Transcutaneous during contact with water conta- minated with cercariae BIIOMPHALARIA SPP	Diarrhoea, cramps Late : portal hypertension Eggs in stools	**Oxamniquine** per os Adult : 1 g Child : 20-40 mg/kg single dose Alternative : **praziquantel** see S. Intercalatum	As above
S. Intercalatum (Central and West Africa) Rare	Transcutaneous during contact with water conta- minated with cercariae PHYSOPSIS SPP	Diarrhoea, cramps Late : portal hypertension Eggs in stools	**Praziquantel** per os Adult : 2.4 g Child : 40 mg/kg single dose	As above
S. Japonicum **S. Mekongi** (SE Asia)	Transcutaneous during contact with water conta- minated with cercariae ONCOMELANIA SPP	Disease often severe : portal hypertension, hepatome- galy, jaundice Epilepsy Eggs in stools	**Praziquantel** per os Adult : 2.4 g Child : 60 mg/kg divided n 3 doses	As above

– Treatment of individuals can be helpful but in a endemic area there is constant reinfection unless preventive measures are taken. The medication is also relatively expensive.

Intestinal protozoa

PARASITE	MODE OF TRANSMISSION	SIGNS	TREATMENT	PREVENTION
Entamœba Hystolitica = Amoebiasis	Direct : person to person contact (dirty hands) Indirect : contaminated water or food	Amoebic dysentery Amoebic liver abscess (fever, large tender liver) Motile forms (not cysts) **must be present in fresh stools to diagnose amoebic dysentery**	**Metronidazole** per os Adult : 1.5 g/d Child : 30-50 mg/d divided in 3 doses x 5 days + **rehydration**	Personal : hand washing, cut fingernails, boil water Community : hygiene, sanitation and supply of clean water, health education
Entamœba Coli Endolimax nana ENTAMŒBA HARTMANI		**Non-pathogenic**	No therapy	
Trichomonas Intestinalis		**Non-paghogenic**	No therapy	
Trichomonas vaginalis	Sexual	Vaginitis Males :usually no symptoms, or urethritis	**Metronidazole** per os Adult : 750 mg/d divided in 3 doses x 5 days or 2 g in 1 single dose	Treat all sexual contacts (even if asymptomatic)
Giardia Lamblia	Direct : person to person contact (dirty hands) Indirect : contaminated water or food	Diarrhoea, cramps, malabsorption Motile forms seen in fresh stools	**Metronidazole** per os Adult : 750 mg/d Child : 10-20 mg/kg/d divided in 3 doses x 5 days Repeat 3 weeks later if necessary	Personal : hand washing, cut fingernails, boil water Community : hygiene, sanitation and supply of clean water, health education
Balantidium Coli (Central America, sometimes Africa)	Direct : person to person contact (dirty hands) Indirect : contaminated water or food	Often asymptomatic Dysentery Parasites in stools	If dysentery, **Metronidazole** per os : as for amoebiasis or **tetracycline** per os Adult : 1.5-2 g/d Child > 8 years : 50 mg/kg/d divided in 3-4 doses x 7 days	Personal : hand washing, cut fingernails, boil water Community : hygiene, sanitation and supply of clean water, health education

6

Therapy for amoebiasis or giardiasis should only be given if trophozoide forms are seen in a fresh stool specimen. Cysts do not necesarrily imply active disease.

Intestinal nematodes (round worms)

PARASITE	MODE OF TRANSMISSION	SIGNS	TREATMENT	PREVENTION
Ascaris lumbricoides (round worm)	Feco-oral (dirty hands)	Often saymptomatid GIT symptoms Anorexia Asthma, allerty **Eggs in stools**	**Mebendazole** per os 200 mg/d x 3 days or 200 mg stat Alternatives : **piperazine** per os 75 mg/kg/d (max 3.5 g/d) x 2 days **pyrantel pamoate** per os 10 mg/kg stat	Personal : hand washing, cut fingernails Community : hygiene, sanitation, sufficient clean water Health education
Ankylostoma duodenalis Nercator americanus	Transcutaneous : bare feet in contact with moist soil contaminated with larva	Allergic symptoms Epigastric pain Anemia **Eggs in stools**	**Mebendazole** per os 200 mg/d x 3 days Alternatives : **pyrantel pamoate** per os : 20 mg/kg stat x 3 days ; **levamisole** per os 2.5 mg/kg stat ; repeat after 7 days	Personal : shoes Community : mass therapy **mebendazole** 200 mg stat Hygiene, sanitation, supply of sufficient clean water Health education
Enterobius vermicularis (pin worm)	Oral (dirty hands) Auto-reinfestation	Often asymptomatic Anal or vulval pruritus Irritability Eggs in stools and around anus ("scotch test")	**Mebendazole** per os 100 mg stat Alternative : **piperazine** per os 50 mg/kg/d x 2 days (max 2.5 g/day)	Personal : hand washing, cut fingernails Community : hygiene, sanitation, sufficient clean water Health education
Strongyloide stercoralis	Transcutaneous : bare feet in contact with moist soil contaminated with larva Auto-reinfestation	Allergic syndrome Epigastric pain Anorexia **Larvae found in stools** (concentration method of Baermann)	**Thiabendazole** per os 500 mg/10 kg stat Take at night. Repeat dose 1 week later. Side effects : nausea, vertigo, vomiting	Personal : shoes Community : hygiene, sanitation, sufficient clean water Health education
Trichuris trichiura (whipworm, tricocephalus)	Feco-oral (dirty hands)	Often asymptomatic Diarrhea in infants **Eggs in stools**	If symptoms : **Mebendazole** per os 200 mg/d x 3 days if diarrhea	Personal : hand washing, cut fingernails Community : hygiene, sanitation, sufficient clean water Health education

Intestinal nematodes (continued)

PARASITE	MODE OF TRANSMISSION	SIGNS	TREATMENT	PREVENTION
Trichinella spiralis Trichinosis (Asia, Africa) Rare	Insufficiently cooked pork meat (non-islamic)	Diarrhea, cramps, fever, myalgiae edema, urticaria **Stools exam negative**	***Thiabendazole*** per os 25 to 50 mg/kg/d divided in 2 doses x 5 days. Alternative : ***mebendazole*** per os 600 to 1,200 mg/d x 3 days, then 1.5 g/d x 10 days (divided in 3 doses)	<u>Personal</u> : cook porkment well <u>Community</u> : veterinary inspection of hords, abattoirs

Intestinal, liver and lung flukes

PARASITE	MODE OF TRANSMISSION	SIGNS	TREATMENT	PREVENTION
Opistorchis – Felinus Clonorchis – Sinensis Liver fluke (SE Asia)	Raw fish	Diarrhea, cramps, allergy, cholecystitis **Eggs in stools**	***Praziquantel*** per os 75 mg/kg/d divisded in 3 doses x 2 days	Cook fish well
Paragonimus Westermani Lung fluke (SE Asia, West Africa)	Raw crab	Cough, heomtysis (mimics TB) **Eggs in sputum**	***Praziquantel*** per os 75 mg/kg/d divisded in 3 doses x 2 days	Cook crab well
Fasciola hepatica et giganta Sheep or liver fluke (Europ)	Watercress	Urticaria Eosinophilia Cholecystitis **Eggs in stools**	***Praziquantel*** per os 75 mg/kg/d divisded in 3 doses x 2 days	Avoid watercress
Others *Heterophyes Metagominus Yokogawai Fasciola Buski* (SE Asia)	Raw fish	Diarrhea, cramps Ofthe asymptomatic **Eggs in stools**	***Praziquantel*** per os 75 mg/kg/d divisded in 3 doses x 2 days	Cook fish well

6

Adult tapeworms

PARASITE	MODE OF TRANSMISSION	SIGNS	TREATMENT	PREVENTION
Tænia saginata *Tænia solium*	Beef (T. Saginata) Undercooked pork (T. Solium)	Non-specific GIT symptoms, irritability. **Segments may be passed with stools.** **Eggs in stools**	**Niclosamide** per os Adult : 1 g, then 1 g again after 1 hour Child : 30 mg/kg stat Alternatives : **praziquantel** per os 10 mg/kg stat **mebendazole** per os 200 mg/d x 4 days	Personal : cook meat adequately Community : veterinary inspection of abattoirs
Hymenolepis *Nana*	Direct (dirty hands) Feco-oral Autoreinfestation	Often asymptomatic Non-specific GIT symptoms **Eggs in stools**	**Niclosamide** per os Adult : 2 g/d x 5 days Child : 30 mg/kg/d x 5 days Alternative **praziquantel** per os 15 to 20 mg/kg stat	Personal : hand washing, cut fingernails Community : water, hygiene, sanitation Health education
Diphyllobothrium latum (Africa, South Asia, Australia, Japon)	Uncooked freshwater fish	Often asymptomatic GIT symptoms Sometimes anemia **Eggs in stools**	**Niclosamide** per os Adult : 1 g, then 1 g again after 1 hour Child : 30 mg/kg stat If anemia : **vitamin B12**	Personal : cook fish

Larval tapeworms

PARASITE	MODE OF TRANSMISSION	SIGNS	TREATMENT	PREVENTION
Hydatid cyst (North africa, South america +++)	Direct : contact with dog (feces) Indirect : via food contaminated by dog	Hydatid cyst of liver of lung	Surgery	Personal : avoid contact with dogs Community : control dogs, do not feed offal to dogs, inspect abattoirs
Cysticercosis (Tænia Solium)	Food contaminated by eggs of T. Solium Autoreinfestation	Nodules in muscle, subcutaneous tissue Ocular and cerebral signs (headache, fits, coma) Eosinophilia	Difficult **Praziquantel** per os 50 mg/kg/d divided in 2 doses x 14 days + **dexamethasone** IM or IV 2 to 3 amp./d Alternative : **thiabendazole** per os (tab 500 mg) 50 mg/kg/d divided in 2 doses x 10 days	Personal : treat infected persons, hygiene, cook meat adequately Health education

Filariasis

 Group of conditions caused by infection with various nematodes, the most common being Wuchereria bancrofti , Brugia malayi , Onchocerca volvulus , Loa loa and Dracunculus medinensis . Adult forms of both sexes live and reproduce in human lymphatics, in the skin or in deep tissues. Their larvæ, microfilariæ, reach the blood or skin and are thus the infective form for biting vectors as well as being the form upon which diagnosis is based.

Transmission is by vector : mosquitoes for lymphatic filariasis (Bancroftian and Malayan), blackflies for onchocerciasis, Chrysops flies for loiasis and tiny crustaceans (Cyclops) for dracunculiasis (Guinea worm).

Clinical features and diagnosis

See table page 121.

Symptomatic treatment

– Inflammatory symptoms :
  acetylsalicylic acid (PO) : 3 g/d divided in 3 doses
  or *indomethacin* (PO) : 75 mg/d divided in 3 doses

– If allergic symptoms develop (e.g. urticaria, pruritis)
  promethazine (PO) : 75-100 mg/d divided in 3-4 doses ; child : 1 mg/kg/d divided in 3 doses
  ou *chlorpheniramine* (PO) : 12 mg/d divided in 3 doses

Antiparasitic treatment

LOIASIS AND LYMPHATIC FILARIASIS

The main drug used is *diethylcarbamazine*, often abbreviated to *DEC*. It is essentially a microfilariacide and may not kill all adult worms. Therapy with DEC should always be supervised as the drug is often poorly tolerated (allergic reactions). Dosages should start low and be increased progressively. DEC is contraindicated during pregnancy. Usual presentation is in 50 mg tablets.

LYMPHATIC FILARIASIS

Adult : commence with 25 mg/d divided in 2 doses (= 1/8 tab x 2/d). Increase progressively by doubling the dose each day until the 5th day, dose is 200 mg x 2/d = 2 tab x 2/d) x 10 days.

Child : 3 mg/kg x 2/d x 10 days, to be reached progressively over 5 days.

A second therapeutical course can be repeated after 10 days.

6

LOIASIS

In this infection *diethylcarbamazine* can cause a fatal encephalitis or allergic shock. Much care is needed. Reinfection after treatment is very common, so if symptoms are mild, it may be better to withold therapy. Dosage can be adjusted to extent of infestation (beyond 50,000 microfilaria/ml blood : +++ caution).
Where treatment considered essential because of severity of infection :
diethylcarbamazine
Adult : 3 mg x 2/d (= 1/32 tab x 2/d) the 1st day increasing progressively till in seven days 200 mg x 2/day (= 2 tab x 2/day) x 21 days.
Child : begin progressively to reach in seven days 3 mg/kg x 2/d x 21 days.

Always give antihistamines in association.
If *promethazine* does not control reactions to treatment, treat with *prednisone* (or *prednisolone*) : 15-30 mg/d in a single dose x 3-5 days, then decrease progressively. If necessary, *dexamethasone* IV or IM : 4-20 mg/kg.

Note : where Loiasis is endemic (West Africa), all treatment with *diéthylcarbamazine*, should commence with 3 mg/kg x 2 days (protocole for Loiasis) whatever form of filaria is being treated. This is to avoid the sometimes fatal complications of inopportune treatment where there is also unrecognised associated loiasis.

ONCHOCERCOSIS

The treatment of choice is *ivermectin* (*Mectizan*®), microfilaricide, 6 mg tablets.
Dose : 150-200 micrograms/kg stat :

     15-25 kg : 1/2 tab
     26-44 kg : 1 tab
     45-64 kg : 1.5 tab
     65-84 kg : 2 tab

The recommended long term management of communities is one dose every 6 months the first year, then a single dose annually.

Contraindications : child < 5 years, pregnant women, women in their first week of breast feeding.

Side effects are due to lysis of microfilaria (allergic manifestations, pain, fever) and respond well to antihistamines and *acetyl salicylic acid.* Rarely orthostatic hypotension occurs but responds to injected corticosteroids (single dose or 1-2 days).
There is no problem with associated filarias even Loiasis.

If *ivermectin* not available : *diethylcarbamazine* in dosage for lymphatic filariosis.

TREATMENT OF MACROFILARICIDES

This should be abandonned as too dangerous.

Prevention – Prophylaxis

– See table on following page.
– Individual chemoprophylaxis for Loiasis is possible, 100 mg *diethylcarbamazine* PO/week in a single dose (or 2 doses of 50 mg/week). It is indicated for non residents going to an endemic zone provided, they are not already infected with Loiasis (risk of serious reactions).

Filariasis *(Tissue roundworms)*

PARASITE	MICRO-FILARIAE	VECTORS	SIGNS	TREATMENT	PREVENTION
Lymphatic filariasis *W. Bancrofti* *Brugia Malayi* (Africa, Asia, Central America)	In blood Nocturnally periodicity	Anopheles, Culex, Aedes (night-biting species)	Acute : adenopathy, lymphangitis, orchitis, fever, headache, asthma, urticaria... Chronic : hydrocele, elephantiasis	Symptomatic : anti-inflammatories and / or anti-histamines Antifilarial : *diethylcarbamazine* Elephantiasis : surgery	Mosquito control : Personal protection Destruction of breeding sites
Liasis *Loa Loa* (West Africa)	In blood Diurnal periodicity	Chrysops (day-biting) ("mangoflies")	May be asymptomatic Pruritus, urticaria, subconjunctival of subcutaneous passage of the worm	None unless symptoms severe : *diethylcarbamazine* with great care	Difficult. Avoid standing in forest in endemic zones Sometimes : mass therapy with *diethylcarbamazine*
Onchocerciasis *Onchocerca Volvulus* (Tropical africa, South America)	In skin (diagnosis from less skin scraping as for leprosy) Non periodic	Simulium spp (day-biting) (blackflies)	Skin : pruritus, lesions, subcutaneous nodules Eyes : uveitis, keratitis, chorioretinitis. End-stage is blindness.	*Diethylcarbamazine* replaced by *ivermectin*, except in pregnant woman, breast-feeding, and child under 5 years : 150 µg / kg single dose	Vector control by insecticide at breeding sites (rivers and streams)
Dracunculiasis *Dracunculus medinensis* (Tropical Africa, Middle East, India, Pakistan)	Ejected by female worm on contact with water	Fresh water crustaceans : Cyclops spp	**Skin ulcer** caused by exit of worm, often secondarily infected Subcutaneous lump Allergic reactions Arthritis	Toilet of ulcers (*dakin* or *chlorhexidine-cetrimide* + *gentian violet*) **Anti-tetanus** prophylaxis **Filarial extraction** (traditional technique Antibiotics if surinfection : *penicillin* or *cloxacillin* per os *chloramphenicol* per os	**Health education** : water filtration or boiling **Protection of water sources** (springs and wells) Vector control (molluscicide)

6

121

Malaria

 Parasitic infection due to protozoa of the genus Plasmodium transmitted by the female anophylus mosquito. There are four plasmodial species : P. Falciparum, P. Vivax, P. Malariae, P. Ovale.

Clinical features

INCUBATION PERIOD

– 9 to 13 days for Falciparum.
– More than 15 days for the other three forms.

PRIMARY ATTACK

Continuous fever + malaise + headache ± gastro-intestinal problems. Consider it in endemic zones.

SIMPLE MALARIAL ATTACK

Shivering, fever ("heat"), sweating, headache, bodyaches. Theoretically, every two days for Falciparum, Vivax, Ovale and every 3 days for Malariae

SERIOUS MALARIAL ATTACK

– *Uniquely due to Falciparum*
  Occurs especially in the non-immune : new subjects, non-residents, children < 5 years, pregnant women, debilitated patients ; or in subjects living in a zone of seasonal transmission.

– *Associated, in varying degrees, with the following clinical signs*
  • Cerebral signs : mental clouding, coma (lasting more than 1/2 hour in children following a convulsion), convulsions (more than 2 times/24 heures in children in the age range for febrile convulsions), delirium, localising signs.
  • Haemolysis (jaundice is rare in children), haemorrhagic syndrome (sometimes C.I.V.D.).
  • Renal signs (rare in children) have bad prognosis : oliguria, anuria.
  • Hypoglycaemia : especially in children and pregnant women.
  • Pulmonary edema : especially in adults ; almost always fatal.
  • Hyperpyrexia : T > 40.5° C.
  • Macroscopic haemoglobinuria.

CHRONIC MALARIA ("MALARIA CACHEXIA")

Due particularly to Falciparum, sometimes Vivax. Usually in children.
Associated with febrile episodes, severe anaemia with pancytopenia, wasting, constant splenomegaly.
Necessary to make repeated staned slides as the protozoa are less numerous.

Diagnosis

Diagnosis is made by presence of protozoa in the blood : thick and thin slides should be made in endemic zones for every fever > 38.5° C.
Note that blood films may be negative, even in a severe attack (pernicious) because of sequestration of parasites in the deep capillaries.

Geographic distribution adapted from W.H.O. (27)

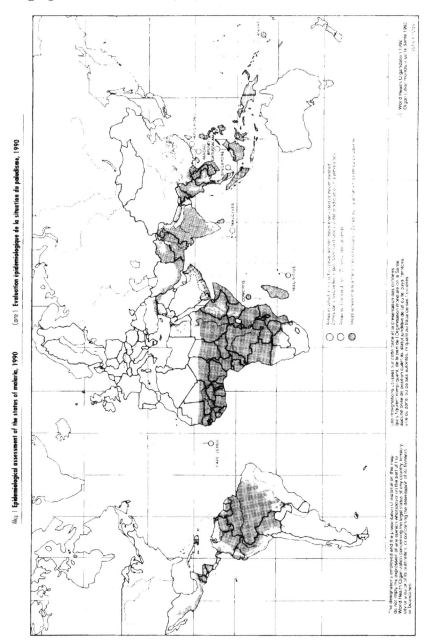

Principal antimalarials

− *Quinine*

- Tablets 100 to 500 mg
  Indications : following IV treatment or a final trial (except in pregnant women in zones of multiresistance).
  Side effects : tinnitus, rarely giddiness, nausea, vomiting.
  Not recommended for prophylaxis.

- Ampoules : available from 60 mg to 300 mg/ml. Never by IV, either infusion or IM (although IM injection canbe given in cases absolute necessity, numerous complications can occur : sciatic nerve paralysis, muscle necrosis, infection).
  Indications : try to reserve quinine by injection for serious cases of malaria.
  No contraindications.

− *Chloroquine (Nivaquine®)*

- Tablets 100 and 150 mg base
  Indications : Vivax, Malariæ, Ovale and uncomplicated attacks of sensitive Falciparum.
  Side effects : pruritis is common in black skinned patients (non-allergic and unresponsive to antihistamines), rarely gastro-intestinal disorders.
  Used for prophylaxis.

- Ampoules 40 and 50 mg base/ml. Never by IV, either IM or SC or infusion.
  <u>Note</u> : the doses for injection are weaker than oral doses.
  Indications : severe vomiting or serious chloroquine-sensitive malarias.
  No contraindications.

− *Amodiaquine (Flavoquine®)*

- Tablet 200 mg
  Active against some chloroquine-resistant varieties. Abandoned because of its toxicity (agranulocytosis, hepatitis).
  Must not be used for prophylaxis.

− *Pyrimethamine-sulphadoxine (Fansidar®)*

- Tablet with 500 mg of sulphadoxine + 25 mg of pyrimethamine, orally

- Ampoule with 200 mg of sulphadoxine + 10 mg of pyrimethamine/ml (= 400 + 20/amp of 2 ml) ; IM (never IV)

Indications : treatment of simple attacks of Falciparum (in zones of intermediate resistance as 1st or 2nd choice.
Side effects : rare but serious : Lyell syndrome, Stevens-Johnson syndrome, agranulocytosis, especially when used for prophylaxis.
Contraindications : pregnancy or breast feeding, children < 2 years (avoid before 5 years).
Sould be abandoned as prophylaxis. Not to be given in association with chloroquine (antagonism) or with mefloquine.

– **Mefloquine** (*Lariam*®) (very expensive)

• Tablets 50 and 250 mg
  Indications : simple attacks of multiresistant Falciparum (as 1st choice in zone III, as 2nd or 3rd choice elsewhere).
  Side effects : giddiness and digestive disturbances are common ; rarely, acute psychosis, encephalopathy with convulsions, transitory but serious.
  Contraindications : epilepsy, history of psychiatric disturbances, avoid in pregnant women.
  Its use for prophylaxis is limited by its side effects.

– **Halofantrine** (*Halfan*®) (very expensive)

• Tablet 250 mg
  Tablets should be taken with a fatty accompaniment
  Indications : simple attacks of multiresistant Falciparum (as 1st choice in zone III, as 2nd or 3rd choice elsewhere)
  Side effects : unobstrusive (pruritis, gastro-intestinal disturbances).
  Contraindications : pregnancy or breast feeding.
  Unusable for prophylaxis.

– **Tetracyclin**

• Tablet 250 mg
  Indications : associated with quinine in areas where the Plasmodium Falciparum is becoming less sensible to quinine (zone III), **use only in severe malaria when the patient is able to swalow**.
  Side effects : nausea, vomiting, photosensitization.
  Contraindications : pregnancy and breast feeding, children < 8 years old.
  Cannot be used as prophylaxis.

6

– **Doxycyclin**

• Tablet 100 mg
  Indications, side effects, contraindications : idem tetracyclin.
  Usable for prophylaxis.

– **Proguanil** (*Paludrine*®)

• Tablet 100 mg
  Only usable for prophylaxis in association with chloroquine including pregnant women and children.
  Very few side effects. No contraindications.

– **Primaquine** : gametocytocide

• Tablet 15 mg
  Indications : avoidance of relapses of Vivax and Ovale. Toxic : methaemoglobinaemia, haemolysis where G6PD deficiency exists (common in Africans, Asiatics and those of Mediterranean origin).
  Contraindications : pregnancy and in G6PD deficiency.
  In practice, few indications (expatriates leaving an endemic zone or where demanded by national rules, especially as resistance to it has been described).

Drug resistance of P. Falciparum

RESISTANCE TO CHLOROQUINE

- Before speaking of resistance, verify :
  - that treatment has in fact been taken,
  - that the correct dose for weight has been prescribed,
  - the absence of important diarrhoea and whether there has been vomiting within one hour of taking medication,
  - the expiry date of the medication,
  - that there has not been under-dosage due to confusion between the expression of the dosage as a chloroquine base and as a chloroquine salt[1].
- There must evidently be a Falciparum positive blood slide on the first and third days of treatment, slides which have been theoretically quantified. There is no chloroquine resistance with P. Vivax, Malariae or Ovale.
- If resistance is suspected, follow the recommendations for the country concerned. WHO has done in vivo testing which is rarely possible in routine practice.
- WHO classifies resistance to chloroquine into 3 types. Schematically :
  - Early and late R 1 : total disappearance followed by reappearance of the parasite
  - R 2 : noticeable fall without diseappearance of the parasite
  - R 3 : parasite level almost unchanged, indeed, increased
- Zones of resistance : see map on following page. There is resistance to chloroquine almost everywhere where Falciparum rages and is more or less frequent depending on the country. Schematically, 3 zones can be distinguished :
  - *Zone I*
    Chloroquine sensitivity retained. Certain West African countries, Central America except for Panama.
  - *Zone II*
    Spreading pockets of resistance, often of low level (R1). East Africa, Northern India, part of West Africa.
  - *Zone III*
    Numerous chloroquine resistant areas of raised level (R2-R3). Multiresistances. South East Asia, part of India and Pakistan, Polynesia, South America.

RESISTANCE TO SULPHADOXINE-PYRIMETHAMINE

- Resistance to *sulphadoxine-pyrimethamine* (*Fansidar*®), although less frequent, has for several years followed closely the distribution of chloroquine resistance. Very extensive in South East Asia and Brazil.

RESISTANCE TO QUININE AND MEFLOQUINE

- Resistance to *quinine* (type R1) and *mefloquine*, also exist principally in South East Asia.

---

[1] NB : the dosage marked on the labels of the boxes is sometimes expressed as the chloroquine salt and sometimes as the chloroquine base. This leads to frequent confusion. Equivalence between salt and base : 130 mg sulphate = 150 mg phosphate or disphosphate = 100 mg base
200 mg sulphate = 250 mg phosphate or disphosphate = 150 mg base

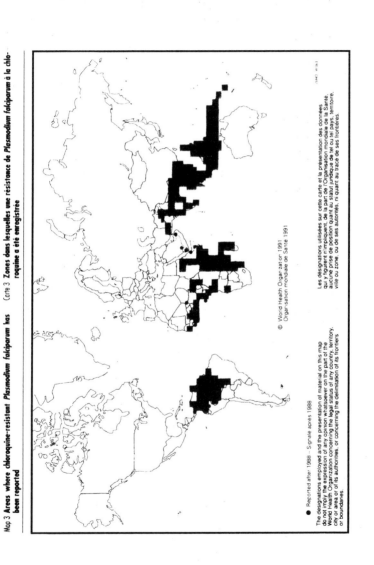

Map 3 **Areas where chloroquine-resistant** *Plasmodium falciparum* **has been reported**   Carte 3 **Zones dans lesquelles une résistance de** *Plasmodium falciparum* **à la chlo- roquine a été enregistrée**

Adapted from W.H.O. (27)

Treatment of primary or uncomplicated attack

– Always use national guidelines. This is essential in countries where drug resistance occurs.

– For *Vivax, Malariæ, Ovale and for Falciparum in zone I* (chloroquine-sensitive) : *chloroquine.*
Adult : 600 mg base then 300 mg base at H6 , D2 and D3
Child : 10 mg base/kg then 5 mg base/kg at H6 , D2 and D3
Or a total of 1.5 g for an adult and 25 mg/kg for a child.

– For *Falciparum in zone II* (intermediate resistance)
   • either *chloroquine* as first choice (eventually 10 mg/kg on D1, D2 then 5 mg/kg on D3, D4, D5)
   and in case of failure, *sulphadoxine-pyrimethamine* :
   Adult : 3 tab in a single dose
   Child : 1/2 tab/10 kg in a single dose
   • or *sulphadoxine-pyrimethamine* as first choice.

Theoretically, *mefloquine* or *halofantrine* are only used in cases of chloroquine and/or sulphadoxine-pyrimethamine failure, with *quinine* as the last recourse. In practice, account must be taken of national guidelines, availability and cost.

– For *Falciparum in zone III*
   • either *mefloquine*
   Adult and child : 15 mg/kg then 10mg/kg 8 hours later ; repeat the dose if vomiting occurs less than one hour after medicament taken.
   In children, if the temperature is lowered before taking the medicine (antipyretics, cold bath), this will decrease the frequency of early vomiting.
   • or (especially in pregnancy) :
   quinine : 30 mg/kg/d divided in 3 doses x 7 days
   in association with *tetracyclin* :
   Adult : 1.5-2g/d x 7 days
   Child > 8 years : 50 mg/kg/d x 7 days
   Tetracyclin is usually contraindicated in pregnancy or breast feeding and children < 8 years, but the vital risk serious malaria makes this a secondary consideration.
   • or *halofantrine* (rarely available becaue of cost)
   Adult : 3 doses of 500 mg at 6 hourly intervals
   Child : 3 doses of 8 mg/kg at 6 hourly intervals
   It should be reserved for cases where resistance has been proven. The ingestion of halofantrine concurrently with fats doubles or trebles its absorption.

Treatment of serious malaria

– *Quinine* as an infusion remains the treatment of choice in every zone. Commence with a loading dose of 20 mg/kg in an isotonic solution (if possible 5 % *glucose*) over 4 hours, then 10 mg/kg every 8 hours (or better, 4 hours with quinine, 4 hours through indwelling venous needle), until such time as the patient can swallow. Then change to oral medication for the remainder of the 7 days.

– SIf the patient has received *quinine* or *mefloquine* in the previous 24 hours without vomiting, a loading dose will not be given (cardiac toxicity).
– If injection is not possible, use *quinine* IM in zones II or III : in the same doses.
– In zone III, complete therapy with *tetracycline*.
– In zone I, *chloroquine* as IM (antero-lateral thigh) or SC can be used in place of quinine. Dosage : 3.5 mg base/kg every 6 hours or as an infusion : 10 mg/kg in an isotonic solution over 8 hours, then 5 mg/kg/8 hours. Transfer to oral therapy as soon as possible. The total dose should be 25 mg/kg.

COMPLEMENTARY TREATMENTS

– Convulsions : *diazepam* IV or IR (see "Convulsions", page 30). For prevention, use with *phenobarbital.*
– Infusion : guard against excessive hydration if not sure of the integrity of renal function. Do not exceed 2,000-2,500 ml/days in adults and 40-50 ml/kg in children, except where there is presenting dehydration which needs to be corrected.
– Transfusion where there is profound or porrly tolerated anaemia (Hb < 5 mg/ml or haematocrit < 15 %). Check for HIV if possible.
– Safe position and nursing in case of coma, nasogastric feeding.
– Record urine output : if < 400 ml/day in adults or 12 ml/kg/day in children, regard patient as anuric. This normally requires fluid restriction. To avoid decreasing the perfusion rhythm and therefore the planned doses of quinine, attempt to initiate a diuresis with *frusemide* IV (ampoule 10 mg/ml, 2 ml) at the rate of 2 ampoules of 20 mg as required (do not exceed 250 mg in 100 ml of 5 % glucose administered over 20-30 minutes in adults ; in children, the dose is 1 mg/kg/inj. repeated every 4-6 hours depending on the evolution).
– Hypoglycaemia : when an doubt, especially in children or pregnant women, give 20-50 ml of 30 % or 50 % *glucose*. Hypoglycaemia often relapses. In practice, in children, the perfusion of 80 ml/kg/day of 5 % *glucose* prevents the hypoglycaemia induced by quinine.
– OAP : *frusemide.*
– Antipyretics as necessary.

6

Specific case : treatment of a simple infection in a non-immune subject (expatriate) and in pregnant women

– *Falciparum infection*

• *In sensitive zones* : *chloroquine.*
either
Adult : 600 mg base then 300 mg base at H6, D2, D3, D4 and D5 (= 2.1 g)
Child : 10 mg base/kg then 5 mg base/kg at H6. D2, D3, D4 and D5 (= 35 mg base/kg)
or
Adult : 500 mg base/d x 5 days (= 2.5 g)
Child : 10 mg base/kg/d x 5 days (= 50 mg base/kg)

- *In resistant zones*
  either ***mefloquine*** : the protocol is the same as for protected subjects except for adults ≥ 60 kg who must take 750 mg, 500 mg, 250 mg at 8 hourly intervals (= 3 tab, 2 tab, 1 tab).
  or ***halofantrine*** : the same protocol as for protected subjects.

- *Pregnant women*
  – In sensitive zones : ***chloroquine***
  – In resistant zones : ***quinine*** (followen by mefloquine if this fails)

– *Vivax , Malariæ or Ovale infections*
chloroquine

Prophylaxis

INDIVIDUAL

– Reserved for expatriates, and depending on the national protocol, for pregnant women.

– Depends on the region to which they are going : see the maps which follow.

– Depends on the length of stay, the season (transmission or not), the presence or absence of resistant Falciparum.

– Protection against anopheles :
  These measures must assume increasing importance :
  • mosquito sprays impregnated with pyrethrinoïd (***permethrine*** or ***deltamethrine***),
  • long sleeves, long trousers and dark clothing at night,
  • repellants,
  • slow combustion anti mosquito coils.

– Information regarding prevention.

– Chemoprophylaxis : does not prevent infection with malaria but may avoid a serious attack. Commence the eve or day of departure and always continue for 6 weeks after return.
  • *In zone I*
  chloroquine : 100 mg base/day, 6 days each week, or 300 mg in a single dose each week.
  • *In zone II*
  chloroquine : 100 mg base/day, 6 days each week, in association with ***Proguanil*** 200 mg/day (in 1 or 2 doses).
  • *In zone III*
  Several possibilities depending on the situation. There is no 100 % efficacious drug, nor any without side-effects.
  either take ***mefloquine*** 250 mg (1 tab) 1 time/week only during the transmission season, or throughout the entire stay if this does not exceed 12 weeks ;
  or where the stay does not exceed 1 month, take ***doxycyclin*** 100 mg (= 1 tab) each day, every day ;
  or take nothing, but carry at all times an effective treatment (***mefloquine, halofantrine, quinine***) to be taken if any symptoms suggestive of malaria appear. Check with microscopic examination of the blood any time this is possible.

– Chemoprophylaxis incorrectly taken means lack of protection.

– Prophylaxis with *sulphadoxine-pyrimethamine* must be abandoned.

COLLECTIVE

It is necessary to carry further the battle against the anopheles mosquito, since mass chemoprophylaxis is no longer recommended (development of resistance, slowing or suppression of protection), except in pregnant women.

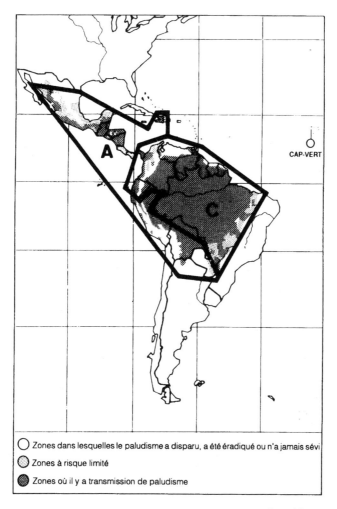

○ Zones dans lesquelles le paludisme a disparu, a été éradiqué ou n'a jamais sévi

◉ Zones à risque limité

● Zones où il y a transmission de paludisme

Adapted from W.H.O. (28)

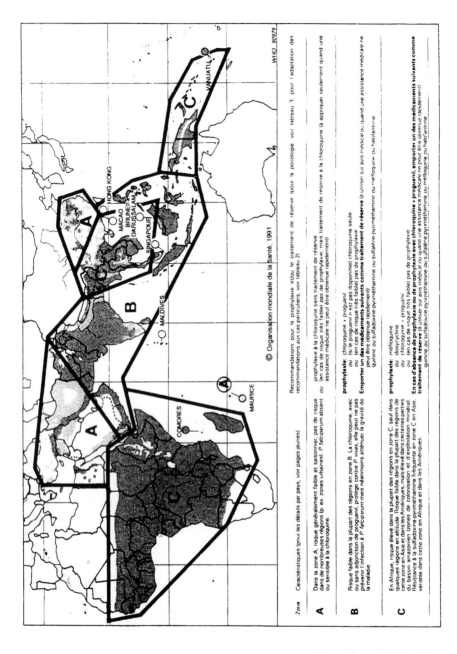

© Organisation mondiale de la Santé, 1991

WHO 90979

Recommandations pour la prophylaxie et/ou le traitement de réserve (pour la posologie, voir tableau 3; pour l'adaptation des recommandations aux cas particuliers, voir tableau 2)

Zone	Caractéristiques (pour les détails par pays, voir pages jeunes)	
A	Dans la zone A, risque généralement faible et saisonnier; pas de risque dans de nombreuses régions (p. ex. zones urbaines). *P. falciparum* absent ou sensible à la chloroquine.	prophylaxie à la chloroquine sans traitement de réserve *ou* (en cas de risque très faible) pas de prophylaxie, mais traitement de réserve à la chloroquine (à appliquer seulement quand une assistance médicale ne peut être obtenue rapidement)
B	Risque faible dans la plupart des régions en zone B. La chloroquine, avec ou sans adjonction de proguanil, protège contre *P. vivax*, elle peut ne pas prévenir l'infection à *P. falciparum* mais néanmoins atténuer la gravité de la maladie.	**prophylaxie:** chloroquine + proguanil *ou* (si le proguanil n'est pas disponible) chloroquine seule *ou* (en cas de risque faible) pas de prophylaxie **Emporter un des médicaments suivants comme traitement de réserve** (à utiliser sur avis médical ou quand une assistance médicale ne peut être obtenue rapidement) quinine ou sulfadoxine-pyriméthamine ou méfloquine ou halofantrine
C	En Afrique, risque élevé dans la plupart des régions en zone C, sauf dans quelques régions en altitude. Risque faible dans la plupart des régions de cette zone en Asie et dans les Amériques, mais élevé dans certaines parties du bassin amazonien (zones de colonisation et d'exploitation minière). Résistance à la sulfadoxine-pyriméthamine fréquente en zone C en Asie, variable dans cette zone en Afrique et dans les Amériques.	**prophylaxie:** méfloquine *ou* doxycycline *ou* chloroquine + proguanil *ou* (en cas de risque très faible) pas de prophylaxie **En cas d'absence de prophylaxie ou de prophylaxie par la chloroquine + proguanil, emporter un des médicaments suivants comme traitement de réserve** (à utiliser sur avis médical ou quand une assistance médicale ne peut être obtenue rapidement) quinine ou sulfadoxine-pyriméthamine ou méfloquine ou halofantrine

Adapted from W.H.O. (28)

Trypanosomiasis

African trypanosomiasis

= sleeping sickness

 – African trypanosomiasis is caused by a flagellated protozoan, which is transmitted to humans by the tsetse fly (*Glossina* spp)
– There are *two species* of the parasite, each having a different geographical distribution :
  • Trypanosoma brucei gambiense (West Africa)
  • T. b. rhodesiense (East Africa)

Clinical features

Clinical manifestations of infections with the two species are similar, except that T. b. rhodesiense infections tend to run a more rapid course.

– *Primary stage* : sometimes a painless chancre appears at site of bite. Incubation period very variable (days to years).

– *Blood stage* : fever, adenopathy, hepatosplenomegaly and facial edema. Presence of trypanosomes in blood and in lymph : gland puncture, blood film

– *Cerebral stage* : chronic meningoencephalomyelitis
  • "Sleeping sickness" : psychiatric, motor and sensory signs
  • Disturbed sleep pattern : hepatosplenomegaly and adenopathy may resolve, blood film becomes negative for trypanosomes, specific serology positive, CSF (raised numbers of lymphocytes (> 5/mm³), raised protein, sometimes presence of trypanosomes, CATT test on serum, Elisa or CSF).

– Other manifestations : T. b. rhodesiense infections may be complicated by a fatal myocarditis.

Prevention

A trypanosomiasis control program must only be conducted in coordination with national health authorities. Consult specialized documents or monographs. Elements :
– Active case detection and treatment.
– Vector control.
– Notification of cases to health authorities (surveillance).

6

Treatment

The choice of regimen is based upon the results of CSF examination. If CSF is normal, the disease is considered to be in the blood stage. Abnormal CSF indicates cerebral involvement.

Table 13 : *Treatment of trypanosomiasis*

Form \ Stage	Blood / Lymphatic	Cerebral
Rhodesiense (T.R.)	**Suramin** IV : 20 mg/kg, do not exceed 1 g/injection For a 50 kg adult : D1 : 0.25 g D2 : 0.5 g D5, D11, D17, D23, D30 : 1g Attain this dosage prgressively.	**Melarsoprol** Amp. IV 3.6 % = 36 mg/ml strict IV only : 1 ml/10 kg/inj., do not exceed 5.5 ml (dry syringe) Begin with : **Suramin** (T. Rhod. or T. Gam.) D1 : 0.25 g D2 : 0.8 g or **Pentamidine** (T. Gam.) D1 : 4 mg/kg then, for a 50 kg adult : D 5 : 2.5 ml D 6 : 3.3 ml D 7 : 3.5 ml D14 : 3.5 ml D15 : 4.0 ml D16 : 4.5 ml D23 to D25 : 5 ml
Gambiense (T.G.)	**Pentamidine** 4 % IM 4 mg/kg, do not exceed 300 mg from D1 to D7 Suramin can also be used except where onchocerciasis is endemic.	**Complementary treatments** Hydration after the injection of melarsoprolol Corticotherapy : **Prednisolone** per os D1 to D7 : 10 mg D8 to D14 : 2/3 initial dose D15 to D21 : 1/2 initial dose Good nutrition, vitamins, iron

Therapy should of course follow national guidelines. Refer also to the WHO monograph (Technical Report Series 739) (29).

Where resistance to melarsoprol develops, use *nifurtimox* according to national guidelines or DFMO.

American trypanosomiasis
= Chagas' disease

☞ Disease caused by Trypanosoma cruzi , transmitted to humans through the feces of infected reduviid bugs, which live in cracks in walls. T. cruzi infects humans via skin lesions (scratches, or bug bite) or mucus membranes, especially the conjunctivæ.

Clinical features

– **Incubation** : 10 to 20 days

– *Acute phase* :
- Chagoma : chancre, often on face
- Unilateral edema of the eyelid and adenopathy
- Persistent fever, generalized adenopathy
- Acute myocarditis : chest pain, CCF
- Hepatosplenomegaly
- Meningoencephalitis : paralyses, convulsions

– **Chronic phase** (after a long latent period) :
- Chronic cardiomyopathy : arrythmias, CCF, angina
- Megacolon, megaesophagus

Diagnosis

– *Acute phase* :
- blood slide : often difficult to find the parasite.
- Xenodiagnosis : examination of the feces of reduvid bugs that have fed upon the patients blood.

– *Chronic phase* : serology.

Treatment *(dispensary - hospital)*

- In spite of progress, treatment for T. cruzi infections is not entirely satisfactory. The drug of choice is at present :
  nifurtimox (PO) : 8 to 10 mg/kg/d divided in 3 doses x 3-4 months.
  - No alcohol during therapy (Antabuse effect)
  - Give **prednisone** ou **prednisolone** (PO) : 1 to 2 mg/kg/day at the same time and taper off gradually.
    NB : this use of corticosteroids is controversial : some sources claim it can exacerbate the disease.
  - Side effects (may be severe) : gastritis, agitation, convulsions, tremor, paræsthesiæ.
  - Contraindications : pregnancy, history of convulsions.

– **benzonidazole** (PO) : 5 to 8 mg/kg/day x 30 days.
  - Side effects : rash, peripheral neuritis

6

Indications for therapy

- Both drugs are active during the acute phase.
  Only **benzonidazole** has an effect during the chronic phase.

- Give supportive treatment of convulsions, CCF and pain.

Prevention

- Mosquito nets.

- Vector control (insecticides) : residual insecticides.

- Improved housing : plastered walls, corrugated iron rooves, cemented floors all reduce the vector habitat (thatch, small cracks in mud).

Leishmaniasis

 Parasitic infection of humans and certain animal hosts caused by flagellated protozoans, Leishmania spp, transmitted by the bite of infected female Phlebotomus sandflies. Two major forms :

- *Cutaneous and mucocutaneous leishmaniasis*
  - Old World, also known as oriental sore (also by many other local names). Occurs in the Middle East, Mediterranean, Ethiopia, India.
  - New World, also known as espundia or mucocutaneous form, occurs in South America and Africa (Ethiopia...).

- *Visceral leishmaniasis, or Kala-Azar*
  - Occurs in the Middle East, Mediterranean, India, East Africa, China, Latin America.

Clinical features

CUTANEOUS LEISHMANIASIS (ORIENTAL SORE) AND MUCOCUTANEOUS LEISHMANIASIS (ESPUNDIA)

- Incubation 2 to 4 months ; single or multiple lesions appear on exposed areas of skin. Starts as a papule, which then extends in circumference and depth to form a crusty ulceration (dry form).
- Wet forms tend to evolve more quickly.
- Lesions tend to resolve spontaneously, leaving a scar.
- Lesion can extend to mucus membranes (mouth, nose, conjuntivæ) and can be very mutilating (mucocutaneous form).

KALA-AZAR

- Persistent fever, pallor, anemia, weight loss, hepatomegaly, splenomegaly ; sometimes adenopathy, diarrhea and hemorrhage.
- Raised ESR, raised gammaglobulins.
- If untreated, is invariably fatal.
- Serology : test for Kala-Azar (direct agglutination, clot Elisa. Always confirm by looking directly for parasites. Serology is of no value in cutaneous forms (false –, false +).

Diagnosis

- By indentification of Leishmania from skin lesions (cutaneous forms), or from blood, bone marrow, lymph nodes or spleen (kala-azar).
- May-Grünwald-Giemsa stain : parasites are intracellular and seen within histiocytes.

6

Treatment

– The main drugs are antimony compounds :
  meglumine antimonate (amp 5 ml = 1.5 g in IM) : 50 mg/kg/d x 10 to 15 days
  sodium stibogluconate (amp. 1 ml = 100 mg in IM or IV) :
  Adult   : 6 ml/day
  Child under 5 years : 2 ml/day
  Child 5 to 14 years   : 4 ml/day
  Duration of 30 days, except with Indian kala-azar which is treated for 6 days only.
  • Idiosyncratic reactions : fever, chills, cough, myalgia and rash. These reactions
    can be fatal so stop therapy if any of these symptoms appear.
  • Therapy must be closely supervised as toxicity may appear late and is serious.
    Signs of toxicity are : fever, chills, cough, rash, polyneuritis, cardiac failure and
    renal failure.

– *pentamidine* (amp. 3 ml = 120 mg in IM) : 2 to 4 mg/kg x 6 injections every 48 hours
  The patient should be supine during and after the injections as they can cause
  either hypoglycæmia or hyperglycæmia.

Indications *(hospital)*

– *Cutaneous leishmaniasis*

Both meglumine antimonate and sodium stibogluconate promote healing but are
not without danger.

  • Systemic *meglumine antimonate* (course of IM injections) can be reserved for
    serious cases.

  • For single lesions, or a small number of small lesions, local therapy can be tried
    instead. Give 1 to 3 ml of *meglumine antimonate* injected around and beneath the
    lesion, to be repeated if necessary.

– *Visceral leishmaniasis*

Either *meglumine antimonate* or *sodium stibogluconate* are given systematically as
described above. Strict supervision is necessary.
In case of poor response or idiosyncratic drug reaction, use *pentamidine*.

Prevention

Vector control and, in some cases, control of animal reservoir.

CHAPTER 7

Bacterial infections

7

Meningitis

 Acute inflammation of the meninges usually of bacterial origin with risk of progressing to encephalitis.

Clinical features

ADULT AND CHILD OLDER THAN 1 YEAR

– Classical meningeal syndrome with fever, meningism, neck stiffness, Budzinski and Kernig's signs positive : the patient lying extended, involuntarily flexes the knees when the neck is flexed or when the legs are raised vertically with the knees in extension.
– If severe : febrile coma, convulsions, localising signs, purpura fulminans.

CHILD UNDER 1 YEAR

Diagnosis much more difficult as classical meningeal signs are often missing. Always think of it in a sick child :
– refusal to eat, fever with diarrhoea, vomiting, drowsiness, plaintive crying, unusual behaviour ;
– generalised or focal convulsions, coma ;
– infant may be hypotonic, neck is often not stiff, fontanelle bulging even when not crying ;

Localising signs :
– purpura may be minimal ;
– slide tests negative ;
– fever may be absent.

Differential diagnosis

Where malaria is endemic, it is vital to consider cerebral malaria (thick and thin slides).

Lumbar puncture

Do lumbar puncture whenever in doubt.

Cerebro spinal fluid (CSF) normal : clear, cells < 5/mm³, proteins < 0.40 g/l (Pandy –).

In meningitis : polymorphs > 500/mm³, proteins = about 1 g/l (Pandy +). *CSF cloudy "rice water" = meningitis.*

Whenever possible, ask for gram staining and direct microscopy for white blood cells.

7

Causative agents

MORE THAN 3 YEARS OLD

- Meningococcus (dry season)
- Pneumococcus (often linked with another focus : pneumonia, RTI)
- Rare other pathogens

2 MONTHS TO 3 YEARS OLD

- Hæmophilus Influenzæ
- Pneumococcus (often linked with another focus : pneumonia, RTI)
- Meningococcus (dry season)
- Rare other pathogens

LESS THAN 2 MONTHS OLD

E . Coli, Listeria, Salmonella, Streptococcus B.

MENINGITIS OUTBREAK

Meningococcus A or C, mainly in Sahel areas, but sometimes elsewhere (Rwanda, Brazil). Outbreaks occur in dry season.

Antibiotic treatment in well equiped hospital

With the exception of *oil based chloramphenicol* IM, the antibiotic utilisable IV (*chloramphenicol, ampicillin, penicillin*) are short acting which necessitates IV injections every 6 hours. If this cannot be done then 1 injection avery 8 hours. The important thing is that injections are given at regular intervals.

Choose the antibiotic effective against the invading pathogen.

MENINGOCOCCUS (GRAM – COCCUS)

- *During an epidemic*

The treatment of choice is *oil based chloramphenicol* IM, 1 single injection, to be repeated 24-48 hours later.
Dosage : 100 mg/kg/injection without exceeding 3 g/injection, giving half into each buttock according to the table.

Age (years)	1	2	6	10	15	
Dose	0.5g	1 g	1.5 g	2 g	2.5 g	3 g

If clinical signs fail to resolve by 3rd day of oil based chloramphenicol, change to *ampicillin* IV.
If necessary, *chloramphenicol* per os can be used : 100 mg/kg/d divided in 3-4 doses x 7 days.

– *When no epidemic*

chloramphenicol IV
Adult : 5-6 g/day
Child : 100 mg/kg/day
in 3-4 IV regularly spaced ; change to oral treatment as soon as possible ; total duration 7 days.

Other treatments are more expensive :
ampicillin IV
Adult : 10-12 g/day
Child : 200 mg/kg/day
in 3-4 IV regularly spaced ; change to oral treatment as soon as possible ; total duration 7 days.
or
penicillin G IV
Adult : 20 MIU/day
Child : 200,000 IU/kg/day
in 3-4 IV regularly spaced ; change to *PPF* IM at the same dose in 1 IM/d (it is not possible to change to oral penicillin V) ; total duration 7 days.

Pneumococcus (Gram + encapsulated diplococcus)

– *ampicillin* IV
Adult : 10-12 g/day
Child : 200 mg/kg/day
in 3-4 IV regularly spaced
or
– *chloramphenicol* IV
Adult : 5-6 g/day
Child : 100 mg/kg/day
in 3-4 IV regularly spaced

In both cases, change to oral treatment as soon as possible ; total duration 8-10 days.

Hæmophilus Influenzæ (Gram – bacilli)

– *chloramphenicol* IV
Adulte : 5-6 g/day
Child : 100 mg/kg/day
in 3-4 IV regularly spaced
or
– *ampicillin* IV
Adult : 12-14 g/day
Child : 200-400 mg/kg/day
in 3-4 IV regularly spaced

In both cases, change to oral treatment as soon as possible ; total duration 8-10 days.

If lumbar puncture is not sterile on 3rd day, treatments can be combined. The chloramphenicol must be given 1 hour after the ampicillin, otherwise antagonism will occur.

7

Management in isolated conditions

- Lumbar puncture if in doubt. If CSF is cloudy, it is bacterial meningitis.

- Begin treatment without delay. Prognosis depends on the speed of initiating treatment.

  • If available : *oil based chloramphnicol* IM (see doses above). Give 2 injections while preparing to transfer to a well equiped centre.

  • If not, *ampicillin* IV or IM, ou *chloramphenicol* IV or IM, or *penicillin G* IV or IM, or *PPF* IM. Give same dosage as for meningococcus.

Supportive therapy

- Ensure adequate nutrition and hydration (infusions, gastric tuve if necessary).

- Convulsions : *diazepam* IV or IR (see "convulsions", page 30).

- Coma : nursing +++ (care against bedsores, care of mouth and eyes).

- Purpura associated with shock : treat shock by restoring blood volume (see "Shock", page 33), plus *dexamethasone* IV :
  Adult : 16-20 mg
  Child : 0,5 mg/kg
  to be repeated as necessary.

Epidemic meningitis

- In risk zones (Sahel in dry season), check weekly incidence of meningitis.

- Decide the critical treshold at which point outbreak is considered an epidemic : either twice the usual weekly incidence (difficult to ascertain) or a level of 20 cases/100,000 inhabitants/weeks (20/100,000/week).

- Inform the local authorities in order to decide public health measures to be instituted.

- Identify the causative meningococcalagent (A or C) by a rapid agglutination test.

- Mass vaccination (vaccine anti A or anti A+C), with all its associated logistic problems, can be decided for the target population : 6 months to 15 years or 25 years. A single injection is sufficient to protect for 3 years. No contraindications. The vaccine is quite stable to heat.

- WHO advises against chemoprophylaxis (sulphonamides, rifampicine). For those who have been in contact with de disease : vaccination, information and supervision +++.

- Treatment : *oil based chloramphenicol* IM (see above).

Pertussis

☞ Whooping cough is a childhood disease characterized by paroxysmal cough and tenacious sputum and caused by Bordetella pertussis. In developing countries it contributes to malnutrition.

Clinical features

Figure 3 : *Clinical course of pertussis*

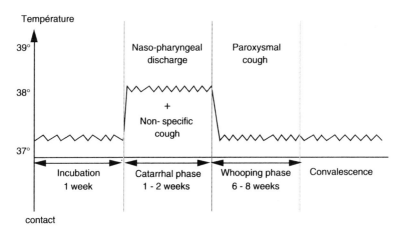

- The cough can recur up to one year after the initial infection.
- Infants less than 3 months may develop apneic episodes or periods of hypoxia (cyanosis) without cough which may be fatal.

COMPLICATIONS

- Anorexia may precipitate protein-calorie malnutrition.
- Subconjunctival hemorrhages, epistaxis, hemoptysis.
- Secondary infections of the upper and lower respiratory system.
- Encephalitis.

Treatment

(dispensary)

– Some authorities recommend antibiotic treatment during the prodromal (catarrhal) stage. This will not alter the course of the disease, but may reduce the period of infectivity and thus reduce transmission.
This is not practical except during epidemics, when all "colds" can be assumed to be prodromal pertussis.
erythromycin (PO) : 50 mg/kg/d divided in 3 doses x 7 days
or
chloramphenicol (PO) : 50 mg/kg/d divided in 3 doses x 7 days

– During the paroxysmal stage, antibiotics are of no use. Advise the mother to ensure adequate hydration, to humidify the air if possible, to remove the tenacious strands of sputum from the oropharynx, and, most important, to continue good nutrition, in spite of the child's anorexia and even if there is vomiting with each coughing spasm (feed the child again after the episode of vomiting).

(hospital)

– Secondary infections : antibiotics PO, IM or IV depending on severity :
ampicillin (PO) : 100 mg/kg/d divided in 3 doses x 5-10 days
or
chloramphenicol (PO) : 50 to 75 mg/kg/d divided in 3 doses x 5-10 days
or
cotrimoxazole (PO) : 40 mg of SMX/kg/d divided in 2 doses x 5-10 days

– Infants less than 3 months of age should be admitted to hospital, if possible, and observed 24 hours a day.

Prevention

– Immunization (part of the routine program).
– During epidemics selective immunization of non-immune infants not manifesting clinical illness who have been in contact with pertussis cases.

Tetanus

 Disease characterized by involuntary muscle spasms, usually fatal if untreated, caused by the tetanus bacillus. The portal of entry is either a wound, or in the case of neonates, the umbilical stump if this has been sectioned with a contaminated instrument. The tetanus victim is usually not immunized (importance of mass immunization programme).

Clinical picture

- Incubation period from 2 to 60 days following wound contamination.
- Trismus, muscle spasms, dysphagia.
- The least stimulus can incite paroxysmal muscle spasms.

Portals of entry

- Dirty wounds.
- Traditional practices during childbirth (e.g. circumcision, ear piercing).
- Surgery.
- Obstetric interventions ; neonatal (2-14 days after delivery) and obstetric forms.
- Unsterile intramuscular injections.

Prevention *(dispensary)*

- **Neonatal tetanus**
  • Sterile instruments for delivery and cutting of the cord.
  • Training of and provision of equipment for traditional birth attendants.
  • Immunization : 2 injections during pregnancy, the first as early as possible (during the first antenatal visit) and the second at least 1 month after the first and no later than 1 month before delivery.
- **Routine immunization of all children** (EPI).
- Correct wound toilet.
- **Prophylaxis** : often tetanus antiserum or booster doses of tetanus toxoid are not readily available. When they are, however, apply the following protocol :
  • Patient fully immunized, having had a booster within the 10 previous years : no further treatment necessary.
  • Patient fully immunized but last booster was more than 10 years ago : give single booster dose of tetanus toxoid (0.5 ml).
  • Patient never fully immunized : equine antitetanus immunoglobulin 250 to 1,500 IU given SC. (Different sources give very different doses.) At the same time start a full course (2 to 3 injections) of tetanus toxoid.

7

– If serotherapy is not available, when there is a dirty wound in an non-immunized or inadequately immunised subject, clean and protect the wound, plus *peni V* or *procaine penicillin* in the usual doses for 5 days.

Treatment (hospital)

– Nurse the patient in a place with minimal sensory stimuli.

– IV fluids : maintain proper hydration.

– Nasogastric tube feeding.

– Equine tetanus immunoglobulin
   Adult   : 10,000 IU SC or IM. Start with a small challenge dose in case of allergic reactions.
   Child   : half the adult dose
   Neonate : 1,500 IU SC or IM
   Equine tetanus immunoglobulin is sometimes given intrathecally : e.g. for neonates, 1,500 IU via either lumbar or suboccipital puncture.

   Reactions to equine tetanus immunoglobulin are treated with :
   dexamethasone (IV) : 4 mg as needed.

– Penicillin G is given in order to eliminate any tetanus bacilli still releasing toxin in the wound :
   penicillin G (IV) : 100,000 IU/kg/d divided in 4 injections

– Control of muscle spasms :
   diazepam (IV) : 1 to 5 mg/kg/d by infusion

   Further sedation if needed :
   phenobarbitone (PO) : 3 mg/kg/d divided in 2 doses by nasogastric tube.

Plague

 – Zoonosis infecting many rodents and transmitted to man by fleas. Plague was formally responsible for pandemics in Europe which caused high mortality.
– Large animal reservoirs persist : South-East Asia, Central Asia, East Africa, Madagascar, South America, USA. Human infection is becoming less common.
– Transmission to humans can be :
  • direct, by the bite of an infected rodent,
  • vector-borne (flea) from a rodent host.
  Both these modes of transmission give rise to sporadic cases only.
  • Epidemics, however, arise when interhuman transmission occurs via flea vectors or, more important, by direct air-borne spread (pneumonic plague).

Clinical features

– *Incubation*
  • 1 to 6 days for bubonic plague
  • several hours to 2 days for pneumonic plague

– *Bubonic form*
  High fever ; painful buboes (adenitis) which are often inguinal (as fleas tend to bite the lower limbs) and produce a sero-sanguineous discharge. Without treatment the case fatality rate is high.

– *Septicemic form*
  A rapidly fatal complication of the bubonic form.

– *Pneumonic form*
  Severe pneumonia with hemoptysis, rapidly fatal. Highly contagious. Occurs either as a complication of the bubonic form or subsequent to primary air-borne pulmonary infection.

Diagnosis

– Identification of Yersinia pestis (staff must take great care not to innoculate themselves accidentally) by :
  • aspiration of a bubo,
  • sputum examination,
  • blood culture.
– Serology becomes positive early.

7

Treatment *(hospital)*

– *Sulphonamides, streptomycin, tetracyclines* and *chloramphenicol* but not the penicillins.

– Usual choice :
streptomycin (IM)
Adult : 500 mg every 4 hours for the first 2 days, then every 6 hours x 5-7 days
Child : 10 mg/kg every 4 hours for 2 days, then every 6 hours for 5 days

– If therapy is begun early the prognosis is good.

– *chloramphenicol* IV can also be used
60 mg/kg/d divided in 3-4 injections x 10 days

Prevention

– If cases are suspected, it is vital to :
• confirm the diagnosis bacteriologically,
• advise local health authorities.

– Where possible plague patients should be isolated.

– Conduct concurrent and terminal disinfection of bedding, clothes...

– Take extreme care when handling exudates and cadavres.

– Give chemoprophylaxis for household contacts and health personnel during the entire period of exposure :
sulphonamides (PO) : 40 mg/kg/d during period of contact
or
tetracycline (PO) : 20 mg/kg/d during period of contact

– Use appropriate insectides to control fleas.

– There is a plague vaccine which is effective for 6 months. Protection begins 7 days after vaccination.

– Long term prevention requires rat control, sanitation and good public hygiene.

Leptospirosis

- A zoonosis due to certain spirochetes also known as Weil's disease. In humans it may cause a febrile illness and acute hepatorenal failure.
- The main reservoir is animal usually rodents (especially the sewer rat), cattle, pigs, dogs, horses, wild animals.
- Infected rats, whether diseased or healthy carriers, excrete leptospiræ in their urine and thus contaminate water and soil (bathing, poor hygiene and sewers...). The portal of entry being either mucous membranes, cuts or scratches on the skin.

Clinical features

- Incubation period of 7 to 10 days. Illness often biphasic. Fever, jaundice, meningism, proteinuria, hematuria and oliguria, hepatosplenomegaly, polyadenopathies.
- Can be associated with :
  • Pulmonary symptoms : cough, pneumonia, hemoptysis ;
  • diffuse haemorrhagic disorder : purpura, ecchymosis, epistaxis... ;
  • severe renal insuficciency : oligo-anuria ;
  • cardiac insufficiency (cardiac collapse).
- The meningeal signs may predominate (the CSF is macroscopically clear with raised lymphocytes and raised protein of 1 g/l). May progress to encephalitis.

Figure 4 : *Clinical course of leptospirosis* (17)

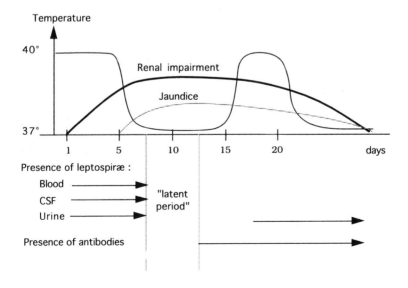

Diagnosis aids

- WBC : frank leucocytosis excludes viral hepatitis.
- Urine : proteinuria, abundant pus cells, hematuria, and easts.
- Diagnosis is confirmed if spirochaetes are found in blood, urin or CSF ; direct examination difficult ; possible with fresh specimen using dark ground microscopy or very low light levels ; otherwise Giemsa stain.
- Serodiagnosis : immunofluorescence or Elisa.

Treatment (hospital)

- Rest.

- Treat fever with *paracetamol* (not acetysalicylic acid, owing to risk of hemorrhagic disease).

- Antibiotics :
  Must be commenced early in the illness if they are to be effective :

  Oral *penicillin* (or IV when serious neurological symptoms). Not IM because of risk of haematoma
  Adulte: 5-6 MIU/d divided in 3 doses x 7 days
  Child   : 100,000 IU/kg/d divided in 3 doses x 7 days

  If allergic :
  tetracycline (PO)
  Adult : 1.5-2 g/d divided in 3 doses
  Child > 8 years : 50 mg/kg/d divided in 3 doses
  or
  erythromycin : same doses as above x 7 jours

Prevention

- Rat control, sanitation and hygiene.
- Avoid swimming in endemic regions
- A vaccine exists for highly exposed individuals (farm workers etc).

Relapsing fever

☞ Relapsing fever or borreliosis is a febrile illness caused by spirochætes and transmitted to humans by lice or ticks. Immunity does not exceed 1 year.
There are two forms of the disease :
- *Louse-borne* caused by Borrelia recurrentis, worldwide distribution and transmitted by body lice. The reservoir is infected humans. The diseases tends to spread in epidemic fashion under conditions of crowding and hardship (e.g. war, refugees, cold and poor hygiene). Pockets notably in Ethiopia, Rwanda and Burundi.
Pockets notably in Ethiopia, Rwanda and Burundi.
- *Tick-borne* caused by many different strains of borrelia which are specific for each geographical region. Reservoir are humans but more importantly infected rodents. Spread by the bites of various ticks and therefore tends to present sporadically rather than epidemically.
Louse-borne fever is often associated with typhus (see Rickettsioses).

Clinical features

LOUSE-BORNE FEVER

Relapsing syndrome of fever, malaise, gastro-intestinal disturbances, jaundice, petechiae, meningism and hepatosplenomegaly.

Figure 5 : *Temperature curve of louse-borne fever*

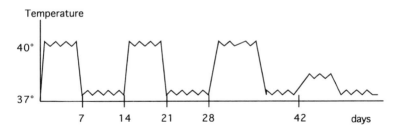

Complications : hepatorenal syndrome, encephalitis, myocarditis, hemorrhage and miscarriage.

TICK-BORNE FEVER

Similar clinical picture.

Diagnosis

Thick and thin blood films during the fever peaks (Giemsa stain).

Treatment *(dispensary - hospital)*

– Same therapy for both forms : either tetracycline, chloramphenicol or erythromycin.

tetracycline (PO)
Adult : 1.5 g/d divided in 3 doses x 7 days
Child : 50 mg/kg/d divided in 3 doses x 7 days

In severe disease, or < 8 years :
chloramphenicol (PO)
75 mg/kg/d divided in 3 doses x 7 days

Single dose of *doxycycline* (PO) is also effective :
Adult : 200 mg
Child : 50 mg

For pregnant women :
penicillin V : 1.2 MIU/d divided in 3 doses x 7-10 days
(beware of procaine penicillin : risk of haematoma).

– Therapy sometimes induces a Herxheimer reaction after the first dose of antibiotics with fever, hypotension and neurological disturbances. *Therapy should therefore be supervised.* Reactions are treated with :
dexamethasone : 20 mg IM or IV
and/or
digoxine (IV) (see "Cardiac failure", page 184)

The following regimen may reduce the chance of reaction :
Day 1 : *PPF* (ou *procain penicillin*) : 400,000 IU (IM)
Days 2 to 7 : *tetracycline* (PO) as above.

Prevention

LOUSE-BORNE FEVER

– Control of body lice : powder body and clothes with an effective insecticide, usually :
1% *lindane*

If resistance, use :
malathion (powder) 1 %
or
propoxur (*Baygon*®)
or
deltamethine (*K-othrine*®)

Use extreme care with these substances (toxic) ; handlers need instructions and supervision. Ask the MOH for guidance.

– In order to be effective the above measure should be applied to the entire population and repeated once after two weeks. This obviously requires good organization.

– Chemoprophylaxis :
doxycycline (PO) : 200 mg / week in single dose during epidemic.
Note that healthy carriers of relapsing fever are at risk of developing a Herxeimer reaction under chemoprophylaxis.

TICK-BORNE FEVER

Control of ticks : insecticides and personal protection.

7

Rickettsioses

☞ – Group of diseases caused by Rickettsia spp, transmitted to humans by an arthropod vector.
– Transmission depends on the presence of :
  • Reservoir of infection : human or animal.
  • Vector : e.g. body lice, often associated with conditions of poor hygiene and sanitation.
  • Crowding : such as in refugee camps.

Table 14 : *The two commonest rickettsioses*

	Louse-borne typhus	**Flea-borne typhus**
Causative agent	R. Prowazeki	R. Mooseri
Reservoir	humans, squirrels, livestock	rats
Vector	lice	fleas
Transmission pattern	epidemic	endemic
Geographical distribution	worldwide (Ethiopia…)	worldwide (Asia, Africa, South America)

There are numerous **other rickettsioses** :
– scrub typhus
– Rocky Mountain spotted fever
– boutounneuse fever
– Q fever…
Their occurrence may be sporadic or epidemic.

Clinical features

– The different forms have a certain common core of clinical features :
  • high fever of sudden onset,
  • severe headache, chills, body pains,
  • macular rash,
  • prostration and coma.

– Evolution of the illness can be cyclical. After 2 weeks, there is a terminal crisis when the signs become more severe then resolve.

– Without therapy, grave and sometimes fatal complications may ensue : encephalitis, myocarditis and hemorrhagic disease.

Diagnosis

Confirmation can only be made by serology.

Treatment *(hospital)*

- Symptomatic for fever, dehydration... **Not aspirin.**
- Antibiotics :
  tetracycline (PO)
  Adult : 1-1.5 g/d divided in 3 doses x 7 days
  Child : 50 mg/kg/d divided in 3 doses x 7 days
  or
  chloramphenicol (PO)
  Adult : 2 g/d divided in 3 doses x 7 days
  Child : 50 mg/kg/d divided in 3 doses x 7 days
- Epidemic louse-borne typhus can be managed by giving a single oral dose of
  doxycycline : 200 mg (but risk of relapse).
- Therapy of typhus should not normally provoke a Herxheimer reaction (see louse-borne relapsing fever) however, in some regions such as Ethiopia, the two diseases may sometimes co-exist in the same patient and a reaction is thus possible.

Prophylaxis

LOUSE-BORNE TYPHUS

- *Control of body lice*
  • Powder body and clothes with an effective insecticide, usually 1% ***lindane.***
  • If resistance, use 1% ***malathion.***
  • Use extreme care with these substances : handlers need instructions and supervision. Ask the MOH for guidance.
  • In order to be effective, the above measure should be applied to the entire population and repeated after two weeks. This obviously requires good organization.
- *Chemoprophylaxis*
  doxycycline (PO) : 200 mg/week in a single dose during epidemic.
  Risk of Herxheimer reaction in asymptomatic carriers of relapsing fever.

FLEA-BORNE TYPHUS

Control of rats and fleas.

7

Brucellosis

☞ – A systemic illness due to the gram negative Brucella. Transmitted to humans from infected cattle, sheep, goats or pigs, either by direct contact with infected tissues or by ingestion of milk.

– Often underdiagnosed, it is probably frequent among animal herders. It tends to occur predominantly among young males, who often have most contact with animals.

Clinical features

– *Incubation* period from 5 to 30 days.

– *Acute brucellosis with septicemia*
Oscillating fever, sweats, flitting pains in the bones, joints and muscles.
Fever then plateaus at 39 to 40°C, with tachycardia.
Defervescence after 10 to 14 days.
Hepatosplenomegaly and generalized adenopathy occur often with a group of nodes gathered around a single larger one.

– *Subacute brucellosis with focalization*
Localized foci of infection that persist and evolve autonomously. But mainly osteo-articular (sternocostal, knee, tibia, spine, sacro-iliac).
Also meningeal and encephalitic foci occur.
Note : brucellosis can minic Pott's disease, osteitis or tuberculosis meningitis.

– *Chronic brucellosis*
Low grade fever, fatigue, vague pains and sometimes infectious foci (such as arthritis).

Diagnosis

– Leucopenia with relative lymphocytosis
– Reaction to intradermal antigen
– Serology : rising titres in Wright's hæmagglutination test or the Rose Bengal card test.

Treatment

ANTIBIOTICS

– *Tetracycline* (PO)
Adult : 2-3 g/d divided in 3 doses
Child > 8 years : 50 mg/kg/d divided in 3 doses

– *Cotrimoxazole* (PO) : tab 400 mg of SMX + 80 mg of TMP
Adult : 6 cp/d divided in 2 doses
Child : 60-70 mg of SMX/kg/d (or 15 mg of TMP/kg/d) divided in 2 doses

– *Streptomycin* (IM)
Adult : 1 g/d in 1 injection
Child : 15 mg/kg/d in 1 injection

– *Rifampicine* (PO)
Adult : 900 mg/d in 1 dose
Child : 20 mg/kg/d in 1 dose

– *Doxycycline* and *chloramphenicol* also effective. Streptomycin can be replaced by *gentamicin*. Never use streptomycin or rifampicine alone.

RECOMMENDED MANAGEMENT

1. First treatment : *tetracyclines* x 6 weeks + *streptomycin* for first 3 weeks.
2. Second treatment : *cotrimoxazole* for 2-3 months.
3. Third treatment : *tetracyclines* + *rifampicine* x 45 days.

INDICATIONS

– *Acute brucellosis*
Use first treatment.

– *Brucellosis affecting bones*
Use first treatment but continue *tetracyclines* a further 45 days or better :
tetracyclines + *rifampicine* for 3 months when possible.

– *Neurologic attack*
Add *rifampicine* to combined *tetracyclines-streptomycin*.

– *Pregnancy, breast feeding or children < 8 years*
Use *cotrimoxazole*, or *rifampicine* + *streptomycin* (if illness does not resolve).

– *Relapse*
Use first treatment if not already tried. If used before, add *rifampicine* or change to *cotrimoxazole* (never use cotrimoxazole and rifampicine together : antagonism).

– *Chronic brucellosis*
Only give antibiotic therapy if persistant focus of infection, otherwise only analysis.

Prophylaxis

– Veterinary measures.
– Washing of hands and clothes after contact with animals.
– Boil milk, avoid fresh cheeses and partially cooked meat in endemic zones.

Typhoid fever

☞ Systemic illness caused by Salmonella typhi, with foci of infection in the lymph and intestine. Transmitted either directly (unwashed hands) or indirectly (contaminated food or water).

Clinical features

- High fever, severe headache, insomnia, prostration, epistaxis.
- Either diarrhea or constipation, abdominal pain, bloated abdomen
- Splenomegaly, rose spots, pulse not in accord with fever.
- Complications (which may appear even during convalescence under therapy) : GIT perforation or hemorrhage, peritonitis, septicemia, myocarditis, encephalitis.
- Leucopenia.
- Widal test (serology) becomes positive around the 8-10th day (for the O antigen non-specific test).
- S. typhi can be isolated from blood or stool during the first two weeks.

Treatment *(hospital)*

- Close observation for complications.
- Treat fever (see pages 26-27) and hydrate (see pages 81-83).
- Oral antibiotics are more effective than IV or IM (since the focus of infection is in the lymph nodes of the small intestine).
  - *First choice*
    chloramphenicol (PO)
    Adult : 2 g/d divided in 3-4 doses
    Child : 75 to 100 mg/kg/d divided in 3-4 doses
    Start initially with half the dose the first day, and increase progressively.
  - *Alternatives* (if resistance or contra-indication to chloramphenicol) :
    ampicillin (PO) (progressive dose)
    Adult : 4 to 6 g/d divided in 3-4 doses
    Child : 100 mg/kg/d divided in 3-4 doses
    cotrimoxazole (PO) (1/2 dose and increase progressively over 3-4 doses)
    Adult : 1,600 mg of SMX/d divided in 2 doses
    Child : 40 mg of SMX/kg/d divided in 2 doses
- If patient cannot take antibiotics by mouth give IV initially but change to oral route as soon as possible.
- Continue treatment for 2 weeks after patient is apyrexial.

Prevention

- Isolation of cases
- Disinfection of excreta with **chlorine solution** 2% or **cresol** 4%.
- Personal hygiene : hand washing and careful food preparation.
- Community hygiene : water, sanitation and health education.

CHAPTER 8

Viral infections

8

Measles

☞ – Also called rubeola and morbilli, it is one of the commonest childhood infectious exanthems. Among children in developing countries it is a serious illness with high mortality, especially when associated with malnutrition. Measles often precipitates acute malnutrition. *Prevention by universal immunization of young children must always be a high priority.*

– Measles is never subclinical, however recent studies have shown that the severity of the disease is related to the infective dose of virus. Crowding tends to increase mortality.

Clinical features

Figure 6 : *Clinical course of measles*

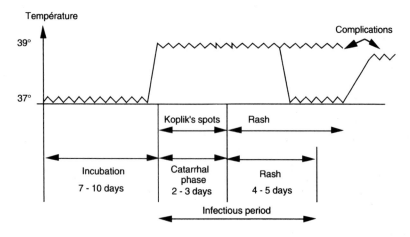

Complications

These must be looked for in all patients.

– Serious signs : persistent fever with darkening of the rash ("black measles") and subsequent desquamation.

– Stomatitis : compromises sucking and eating.

– Laryngitis : distinguish a benign prodromal laryngitis from that due to a secondary infection, which may be severe.

– Croup and otitis media.

- Bronchopneumonia : usually severe ; gram negatives or staphylococcus.
- Diarrhea : either due to virus or from a secondary infection.
- Vitamin A deficiency : keratoconjunctivitis. Measles increases the con-sumption of vitamin A and often precipitates xerophthalmia.
- Encephalitis : caused by the measles virus itself ; it occurs on about the 5th day of the rash.
- Malnutrition : precipitated by anorexia, stomatitis, fever, vomiting, diarrhea and other complications. Also important are frequent harmful cultural taboos that impose fasting upon a child with measles.

Treatment

(dispensary)

- Active case-finding during epidemic, if practical (home visits).
- Treat the fever (see pages 26-27).
- Keep well hydrated (see pages 81-83).
- Observe closely for complications.
- Give prophylaxis against conjunctivitis : drops or ointment.
- Give prophylaxis against xerophthalmia : *vitamin A*
  Infants   : 100,000 IU in single dose on day 1, day 2 and day 8
  After 1 year : 200,000 IU in single dose on day 1, day 2 and day 8
- Encourage good oral hygiene (see page 75).
- Maintain adequate protein-calorie intake : educate mothers (especially if cultural taboos against feeding exist), continue breast feeding, provide supplementary feeding if available (but do not admit to a feeding center until after infectious period).
- Antibiotics are often given prophylactically :
  penicillin V(PO) : 100,000 IU/kg/d divided in 3 doses x 5 days
  or
  cotrimoxazole(PO) : 60 mg of SMX/kg/d divided in 2 doses x 5 days

(dispensary - hospital)

- Treat secondary infections with antibiotics :
  ampicillin : 100 mg/kg/d divided in 3 doses
  or   per os, IM or IV
  chloramphenicol : 75 mg/kg/d divided in 3 doses   according to gravity
  or   x 7-10 days
  cotrimoxazole : 60 mg of SMX/kg/d divided in 2 doses

8

– Give supportive therapy for meningoencephalitis :
Adequate hydration, good nursing, nasogastric feeding and control convulsions
with *diazepam* (see pages 30-31).

Prevention

– Education of mothers must be part of the MCH program.

– Immunization :

- A single injection gives good protection. Ideally should be given at the age of
9 months, but is often given later.

- Measles immunization is one of the highest priorities in refugee settings and
other situations where crowding, poor hygiene and precarious nutritional status
combine to encourage both transmission and the emergence of complications.

- There is an Oxfam / WHO measles immunization kit that is designed for
emergency situations. Newly arrived refugee populations should be immunized
during the first days of the emergency and all new arrivals should be
immunized on entering. The target age-group is children from 9 months to
12 years (up to 5 years if resources are very scarce).

Poliomyelitis

 – Acute infection due to the three strains of poliovirus affecting infants and young adults. It is endemic in developing countries but may occur in seasonal epidemics among non-immune persons. Transmission is feco-oral.
– Polio should disappear when immunization is universal. A very high proportion of cases are asymptomatic and these healthy carriers are the reservoir of infection : only 0.1% of infections give rise to paralysis. Polio occurs endemically in developing countries but seasonal epidemics can also occur.

Clinical features

– Febrile flu-like illness, often with diarrhea.
– Sometimes aseptic meningitis.
– Paralytic forms : paralysis is of sudden onset (often noted on waking in the morning), asymmetrical and hypotonic. It is associated with fever, hyporeflexia, risk of respiratory paralysis and eventual muscle wasting.

Treatment (hospital)

Is supportive only :
– Treatment of the fever and diarrhea.
– Rest, nursing care for paralytic cases.
– Physiotherapy once signs have stabilized.

Prevention

– Immunization with live attenuated trivalent oral polio vaccine (OPV) with first dose at birth (new WHO recommendation) and then 3 more doses at the 6th, 10th and 14th weeks.
– Salk injectable killed vaccine at the 6th, 10th and 14th weeks.
– Theorically, boosters 1 year later and 5 years after that.

8

Public health measures

Community-level management :
– A paralytic case signifies that the virus is in circulation.
– Confirm the diagnosis serologically (rising titres).
– The immunization status of the community should be determined : date of the most recent program, coverage...
– If necessary, plan and implement a mass immunization program for children aged from 3 months to 5 years and carry out an "outbreak investigation".

Arbovirus diseases

 Viral illnesses that usually have an animal reservoir and are trans-mitted to humans by mosquito vectors. They occur either sporadically or in epidemics.

Clinical features

Different viruses have different manifestations ; however there are four main syndromes :
- Flu-like viral illness : e.g. dengue fever (SE Asia and the Pacific).
- Encephalitis : fever, neurological signs, convulsions, coma, sometimes meningism with a clear CSF. E.g. Japanese B encephalitis (SE Asia).
- Hepatorenal syndrome : fever, jaundice, oliguria, albuminuria, sometimes hemorrhages. E.g. yellow fever (West Africa, South America).
- Hemorrhagic fever : clinical picture of severe dengue fever plus shock and hemorrhagic manifestations in skin and mucosæ. E.g. dengue hemorrhagic fever (usually only seen in children in SE Asia) ; also diseases such as Lassa fever, Ebola and Marburg v:rus, which have caused fulminant and deadly epidemics in Africa.

Treatment (hospital)

There is no causal therapy. Treatment is supportive.

Prevention

- Immunization : only a vaccine for yellow fever is available. A single injection protects for 10 years.
- Personal protection : mosquito nets, adequate clothing.
- Vector control : sanitation, destruction or management of vector breeding sites (e.g. domestic refuse, water containers for urban Ædes ægypti, the vector of yellow fever).
- Epidemic management :
  • Confirm the diagnosis : virological and serological studies in the nearest reference laboratory. One should collect detailed clinical and epidemiological information.
  • Alert the local authorities.
  • Plan control measures with the local authorities : vector control, public education and an immunization campaign.

Rabies

☞ Viral zoonosis transmitted to humans in the saliva of an infected animal. Innoculation can be by :
– *bite* : dog, cat, wild animal, vampire bats (South America),
– *licking open skin lesions* : cats, dogs, goats…

Principles of preventive therapy

– The risk of exposure to rabies is higher in developing countries because of the high prevalence of the disease in stray animals.

– Clinical rabies in humans is invariably fatal but can be prevented with vaccine and antiserum after exposure.

– The incubation period in humans is from 2 weeks to several months depending on the severity and site of innoculation.

– An infected animal sheds rabies virus in its saliva before it develops signs of disease (14 days for dogs and cats).

Table 15 : *Treatment according to animal exposure* (3)

Guide to prophylaxis after exposure

The following recommendations are self-explanatory. The decision to treat depends on the type of animal involved, the circumstances fo the bite, the vaccination status of the victim and the prevalence of rabies in the area. In in doubt, consult the local health authority.

Type of animal	Condition of animal at time of exposure	Treatment vaccination or serum + vaccination
Domestic cat or dog	Normal and can be observed for 10 days	None unless anima develops rabies
	Abnormal / ? rabies	Yes
	Unknow	Yes
Carnivorous wild animals	Consider the animal has rabies unless there is biological proof to the contrary	Yes
Other animals (cattle, rodents)	Consider case by case Usually consider animal is free of rabies unless there is biolo-gical evidence to the contrary	Yes according to case

8

– There are two types of exposure :

- *Benign* : contact of saliva with scratches on the skin ; minor bites on the trunk or proximal limbs.

- *Serious* : contact of saliva with mucus membranes ; bites on the face, head, neck, hands, feet, genitals ; and bites from a wild animal.

Management of a person exposed to rabies *(dispensary)*

AFTER BITE

– Wash wound with soap, rinse, then dry thoroughly.

– Clean wound with *chlorhexidine-cetrimide* or other antiseptic and do not suture.

– Give tetanus prophylaxis.

– Capture and observe the animal for 15 days.

– Treatment :
- *antirabies serum* (Pasteur) : prepared from horse immunoglobin.
- *rabies vaccine* (Pasteur) : human diploid cell vaccine (HDCV).

– *Note* : the old vaccines (e.g. duck embryo) require several injections (7-14) and have allergic and neurological complications.

INDICATIONS FOR VACCINATION

– Depends on the condition of the animal at the time of the bite and after 15 days.

– There are two regimens :

- *Benign exposure* : **simple rabies vaccination**
1 dose (SC or IM) on day 0 (the start of the schedule), day 3, day 7, day 14, day 30 and day 90.

- *Serious exposure* : **serum + vaccination**
Day 0 (as soon as possible after the bite) : give serum 20-40 IU / kg IM
Then Day 1, 8, 15, 30 and 90 : give 1 dose of rabies vaccine.

Preventive measures for exposed personnel

Personnel who may be exposed to rabies (e.g. veterinarians, technicians) should be given 3 doses of rabies vaccine (HDCV) on days 1, 7, 21 or 28 and a booster dose after 6 months.

Table 16 : *Rabies prophylaxis*

Nature of exposure	Condition of animal		Prophylaxis
	At time of exposure	14 days later	
1. *Saliva in contact with skin, but not skin lesions*	Healthy	Healthy Rabid	No therapy
	Suspect	Healthy Enragé	No therapy
2. *Saliva in contact with skin that has lesions (scratches...), minor bites or trunk or proximal limbs*	Healthyn	Healthy Rabid	No therapy Vaccination
	Suspect	Healthy	Vaccination : stop course if animal healthy after 5 days
		Rabid	Vaccination
		Rabid or unknow (wild animal or domestic animal cannot be observed)	Vaccination
3. *Saliva in contact with muosa, serious bites (face, head, fungers or multiple bites)*	Domestic or wild animal, rabid or sus-pect, or animal cannot be observed		Vaccination Antirabies serum Stop therapy if still healthy after 5 days

W.H.O. (30)

8

Hepatitis

☞ Several viral infections come under the heading viral hepatitis, each having its own epidemiology, clinical characteristics, immunology and prognosis.
Hepatitis A, B, D and E occur in the tropics. The geographic distribution of hepatitis C is not yet known. All hepatitis, when they resolve, result in life long immunity, but not shared immunity.
The old terminology, non A-non B (A like-B like) has now been changed to hepatitis C and E. The "defective" virus D needs the presence of virus B to develop.
Principle characteristics are summarized in table 17, page 171.

Clinical features

ACUTE HEPATITIS

Nausea, fever, fatigue, abdominal discomfort, followed by the appearance of jaundice having an element of biliary obstruction, dark urine and stools more or less pale.

SUBCLINICAL INFECTION

Mild or anicteric infection is the most common but exposes the sufferer to the same risks.

FULMINANT HEPATITIS

Severe acute infection that leads to necrosis and liver failure. It is associated with high mortality.

CHRONIC ACTIVE HEPATITIS

May lead to cirrhosis and eventually hepatoma.

Treatment

– Symptomatic : rest, caution in prescribing analgesics (eg. acetyl salicylic acid, paracetamol), correct but not specific diet and hydration.
– Avoidance of corticosteroid therapy. Several medications are contraindicated.

Vaccination

Plan to include anti-B vaccine in the Expanded Program of Immunization (EPI).

Table 17 : *The different forms of viral hepatitis*

	HEPATITIS A	HEPATITIS B	HEPATITIS C	HEPATITIS D	HEPATITIS E
Incidence	Childhood	Young adult	Young adult	Young adult	Young adult
Incubation period	2-6 weeks	4-30 weeks (average 10 weeks)	2-25 weeks	Co-infection B-D : consequence of hepatitis B Superinfection of carrier chronic B : about 5 weeks	2-8 weeks
Infectious period	Precedes signs Brief : < 10 days after the appearance of jaundice. Maximal at the end of incubation period	Precedes signs Lasts whole of active period Can persist in chronic carriers	Precedes signs Duration poorly understood, seems identical with virus B. Could persist beyond normalisation of transaminases	Precedes signs Duration poorly understood. Seems identical with virus B	Precedes signs Duration poorly understood (10-15 days after the appearance of jaundice)
Transmission	Faeco-oral Contaminated water and food Rarely transfusion	Blood and its derivatives Sexual. Contaminated blood products Vertical (mother to neonate)	Blood and its derivatives Sexual : weak Contaminated blood products : weak Probably vertical	Blood and its derivatives Sexual (especially homosexual). Contaminated blood products Vertical possible	Faeco-oral Contaminated water and food
Fulminant forms	0.2 - 0.4 %	1 to 3 %	Rarer than hepatitis B	Much more common in the case of superinfections in a carrier of B than in the case of co-infection B-D	Mortality 10-40 % in pregnant women
Long term prognosis	No chronic forms	Chronicity : 0.2-10 % of which 5-15 % progress to cirrhosis Hepatoma possible	Chronicity : up to 50 % of which 10-25% progress to cirrhosis Hepatoma possible	Chronicity : 2-5 % of co-infections B-D and > 90% of superinfections in a B carrier (rapid cirrhosis)	No chronic forms
Personal prevention	Non-specific immunoglobulin injections	Specific immunoglobulins anti HBS Safe sex (condoms)	Anti HBS immunoglobulins can be effective	Same as for hepatitis B (virus D can only develop with B)	Specific immunoglobulins for pregnant women
Vaccination	New vaccine	Anti-hepatitis B	Non existant	Anti-hepatitis B	Non existant
Community prevention	Hygiene, sanitation	Problems of transfusion (limitation, detection in blood banks), disposable transfusion materials			Hygiene, sanitation

8

A.I.D.S. and infection by VIH

☞ AIDS, or Acquired Immune Deficiency Syndrome,is the most serious form, the end stage of infection by HIV (Human Immune-deficiency Virus). The virus attacks the immune system by infecting and then destroying the T4 lymphocytes.

Infection by HIV develops as a function of time, schematically :

– *Incubation period*
From infection by the virus to the appearance of specific anti-HIV antibodies, lasts on average 6 weeks, sometimes marked by a non specific febrile syndrome (pseudo influenza syndrome).

– *Asymptomatic period*
This is the seropositive phase which can last years. The diagnosis depends on the detection of specific anti-HIV antibodies in the blood. On average, 50 % of seropositives progress to AIDS in 10 years (with actual decline).

– *Symptomatic period*
The immune deficiency syndrome is manifested clinically, it is the clinical AIDS phase. The pre-AIDS syndrome which was at a certain time defined by the term ARC (AIDS-related complex), is les and less recognised as a physiopathological entity. This is why there is no mention made of it here.

Epidemiology

HIV / AIDS infection is pandemic, occurring in epidemic form on 5 continents : however, not all populations are uniformly affected in one country or another or in the midst of the same country.

PREVALENCES

– *Seropositives*
In April 1991, WHO estimated that 8-10 million adults in the world had been infected by the virus since the beginning of the epidemie. Of these more 60 % were in Sub-Saharan Africa and around 1 million were children.

– *Clinical AIDS*
In April 1991, WHO estimated the number of clinical AIDS cases to be 1.5 million since the beginning of the epidemie (345,000 notified cases), 500,000 cases were children.

– *Serotypes*
Two serotypes have been identified : HIV 1 and HIV 2.
HIV 1 is the most widespread.
HIV 2 is particularly found in West Africa and spreads less rapidly than HIV 1. However, the modes of transmission and the clinical picture do not differ from one serotype to the other.

HIV TRANSMISSION

- *Sexual transmission*
During improtected homosexual and heterosexual relations. 70 % of the world's HIV infections result from heterosexual transmission.

- *Blood transmission*
By transfusions, contaminated surgical instruments, contaminated syringes and needles, by contact of even a minimal wound with contaminated blood (surgery or childbirth delivery without gloves, injury or prick with a needle or instruments contaminated with infected blood).

- *Materno-fœtal transmission*
During pregnancy or delivery.
Note : transmission breast feeding is possible : nevertheless, the relationship between benefits and risks is such that WHO continues to recommend this form of feeding.

- *HIV is not transmitted* by saliva, mosquitoes, air, water, food, skin contacts, clothing, cooking utensils, the movement of general daily life.

Table 18 : *Geographic distribution and principal modes of transmission*

	TRANSMISSION	COUNTRIES WITH MAJOR INCIDENCE (countries having a system of surveillance, known data)
Africa	Heterosexual +++ Perinatal ++ Transfusions +	East and Central : Kenya, Uganda, Rwandi, Burundi, Zambia, Tanzania, Malawi, Zaire, RCA... West : Ivory coast, Congo, Guinea-Bissau...
Asia	Heterosexual +++ Drug-addict +++ Transfusions + Perinatal +	Thailand, India... Others...
Latin America The Carribbean	Homosexual +++ Heterosexual +++ Drug-addict ++ Transfusions + Perinatal +	Brazil, Mexico, Haïti... Others...
Western Europe Australia North America	Homosexual +++ Drug-addict +++ Heterosexual + Perinatal +	USA, France, Switzerland, Denmark...

8

Projections

– <u>Groups at risk</u> : heterosexual transmission is the origin of 70 % of cases of infection in 1991, the groups at risk for the decade 1990-2000 will be heterosexual populations with multiple partners.
– <u>Geography</u> : 90 % of cases will survive in developing countries, Sub-Saharan Africa, Asia and Latin America.

Clinic factors

Table 19 : *Clinical definition of AIDS – WHO (Bangui, 1985-1986)*

ADULT	CHILD
Major signs – Loss of weight ≥ 10 % – Chronic diarrhoea ≥ 1 month – Persistant fever ≥ 1 month	*Major signs* – Loss of weight or growth retardation – Chronic diarrhoea ≥ 1 month – Persistant fever ≥ 1 month
Minor signs – Persistant cough ≥ 1 month – Generalized pruritic dermatitis – Relapsing herpes zoster – Oropharyngeal candidiasis – Progressive, generalized, chronic hepatic infection – Generalized lymphadenopathy	*Minor signs* – Persistant cough – Generalized dermatitis – Repeated minor infections – Oropharyngeal candidiasis – Generalized lymphadenopathy – Confirmation of maternal HIV infection
In the absence of cancer severe, malnutrition or another recognized cause of immunodepression, AIDS is defined : – By the presence of at least 2 major signs and at least 1 minor sign – Or by the presence of a generalized Kaposi sarcoma – Or by the presence of cryptococcal meningitis	In the absence of cancer severe, malnutrition or another recognized cause of immunodepression, AIDS is defined : – By the presence of at least 2 major signs associated with at least 2 minor signs
Performance of the definition : This varies according to the clinical context and the prevalence of AIDS in each country. It must therefore be notified by these. – Average sensitivity = 60 to 70 % – Average specificity = 80 to 90 %	Performance of the definition : The paediatric definition of AIDS is much less sensitive and specific than that for adults, but is at present the only one utilisable.

This exclusively clinical definition is intended for developing countries lacking laboratory facilities (culture and/or histology). It is, above all, an indispensable tool in the surveillance of AIDS (notification of cases) and an elaborate clinical tool permitting clinicians to make a diagnosis with the maximum precision.

Table 20 : *Clinical forms of AIDS in Africa*

GENERAL MANIFESTATIONS

Persistant fever without specific characteristics
Excessive sweating frequently noted
Anorexia is very frequent
Early weakness (asthenia)
Loss of weight is almost constant
Cachexia

SYSTEMATIC MANIFESTATIONS

Digestive forms (50 % of cases)
Diarrhoea (70 to 80 % of cases)
Oesophageal candidiasis

Respiratory system
Pneumocystosis
Tuberculosis
Kaposi's sarcoma
Pneumonopathies of CMV
Minor bacterial infections

Neurological/psychiatric forms
Violent cephalitis, resistant to analgesics
Meningo-encephalitic syndrome
(cryptococcosis, tuberculosis,
toxoplasmosis, HIV encephalitis)
Neurological deficit syndrome
Psychiatric syndrome (confused
behavour, hallucinations)
Peripheral myopathy and neuropathy

Cutaneomucous forms (50 % of cases)
Pruritis
Buccal and cutaneous candidiasis
Buccal leucoplasia
Other mycoses
Herpes zoster (relapsing ++)
Kaposi's sarcoma
Chronic herpes

Lymphatic forms
Generalized lymphadenopathy

Others
Extrapulmonary tuberculosis
Generalized atypical mycobacterioses

Serological diagnosis of HIV infection / AIDS

In conditions in the field, the diagnosis of HIV infection in the asymptomatic adult can only the serological, i.e. the presence of specific anti-HIV antibodies in the blood is the sign of infection.

Table 21

	INDICATIONS
Simple test (rapid) = small series of blood samples	Blood samples before transfusion Epidemiological supervision Voluntary and confidential blood samples
Elisa = large series of blood samples	Blood samples before transfusion Epidemiological supervision Voluntary and confidential blood samples
Western Blott = reference laboratory	Epidemiological supervision Confirmation of seropositivity

In practice, the serological diagnosis of *suspected AIDS* is of no therapeutic interest. It can be justified for certain suggestive clinical tables of AIDS, but without satisfying the criteria of WHO clinical definition.

PRINCIPLES OF SEROLOGICAL DIAGNOSIS

To prescribe a serological test and announce the result *negative or positive,* for an HIV test, it must be combined with all the following conditions :

1. The patient must have received appropriate information about the consequences of a positive result and have given prior permission to be tested for anti-HIV antibodies.

2. Positive results from a blood sample must be confirmed by Western-Blott.

3. The seropositive individual must be able to benefit from further medical care and advice +++.

4. Confidentiality.

Treatment of HIV infection and AIDS

ANTIRETROVIRAL THERAPY

The only molecule in current commercial production is AZT (Azidothymidine). Its cost (2,000 - 3,000 US$/year) and the necessary techniques for therapy prevent, at present, its general use in developing countries.

TREATMENT OF OPPORTUNIST OR ASSOCIATED INFECTIONS (WHO GUIDELINES)

See tables 22a, 22b and 22c on the following pages.

Table 22a

SYNDROME	DEFINITION AND ETIOLOGY	GUIDELINES FOR MANAGEMENT	TREATMENT	
Chronic diarrhoea (bloody or not)	More than 3 liquid stools/day either permanent or in episodes of more than one month *Infection*: Cryptosporum Isospora Giardia Shigella Salmonella Entamoeba hyst. *Neoplasia*: Kaposi Lymphoma *Idiopathic*: (HIV?)	1. Dehydration prevention ++++ treatment ++++ cf chap. 3 "Diarrhoeas" 2. Nutrition ++++ 3. Examination of stools Make at least 3 examinations	1. Clinical/lab. suspicion = bacterial infect. *cotrimoxazole* 480 mg : 2 tab x 2/day for 5 days If no response : *metronidazole* 500 mg x 3/day for 7 days 2. Clinical/lab. suspicion = parasitic infect. *metronidazole* 500 mg x 3/day for 7 days If no response: *cotrimoxazole* 480 mg : 2 tab x 2/day for 5 days 3. No clinical/lab. orientation = empirical treatment *cotrimoxazole* and/or *metronidazole* *mebendazole* 500 mg x 3/day for 7 days (Strongyloides) *erythromycin* 2 g/day for 5 days (Campylobacter)	If no improvement (and no contra-indications = bloody diarrhoea) : symptomatic treatment : *loperamide* 4 mg initial dose + 2 mg after each liquid stool (max. 16 mg/day) If after improvement the diarrhoea recurs within 4 weeks : recommence treatment for 6-12 weeks
Buccal plaques	Presence fo white deposits on an erythematous base on the bucal mucosa, the dorsum of the tongue, the gums, the palate or the pharynx Candida Albicans	1. Lab. examination if necessary to confirm 2. Look for dysphagia, pain on swallowing = suspect oesophageal candidiasis	1. Moderate buccal candidiasis Application to totale area of *gentian violet* 1 % 2 x/day or *nystatin* per os 500,000 IU x 3/d for 7 days 2. Severe buccal candidiasis/resistant local treatment *ketoconazole* 200 mg x 2/d for 7 days or *fluconazole* 50 mg/d for 7 days 3. Oesophageal candidiasis *ketoconazole* 200 mg x 2/d for 14 days or *fluconazole* 100 mg/d for 7 days	If no improvement, differential diagnosis leucoplasia CMV oesophagitis herpetic infection The duration of treatment is only suggested ; it must be followed up to the disappearance of signs and symptoms

8

Table 22b

SYNDROME	DEFINITION AND ETIOLOGY	GUIDELINES FOR MANAGEMENT	TREATMENT	
Respiratory conditions	Cough and / or thoracic pain and / or persistent dyspnoea in patient suffering from symptomatic HIV infection *Infection:* CMV progene, Toxoplasmosis, Mycobacterium tuberculosis, Mycobacterii, Pneumocystis carinii, Endemic mycoses, others *Neoplasia :* Kaposi's sarcoma Lymphoma *Other :* Interstitial pneumonopathy lymphoides	1. Examination of sputum 3 especimens looking for Koch's bacillus 2. X-Ray chest (lungs) TB = hilar adenopathies and / or mediastinal + infiltration of middle or inferior lobes (cavities and infiltration of superior lobes are rare in HIV sufferers) *Pneumocystosis* = bilateral interstitial infiltrations	1. If sputum examination positive or X-Ray of thorax suggests tuberculosis Antitubercular treatment (cf chap.2) 2. If sputum examination negative and X-Ray of thorax suggest a pyogenic infection *penicillin* 250 mg 2 tab x 3 / d for 10 days o *ampicillin* 500 mg 2 tab x 3 / d for 10 days 3. If sputum examination negative and X-Ray of thorax suggest a pneumocystosis *cotrimoxazole* 480 mg 3-4 tab x4 / d for at least 14 days and preferably 21 days or *pentamidine isothionate* 3-4 mg / kg / day	The risk of severe reaaction to *thioacetazone* is increased in the patient with HIV infection If no improvement by day 3, change the antibiotic ex. *cotrimoxazole* 480 mg 2 tab x 2 / d for 10 days Improvement from day 7, secondary prophylaxis is recommended ex. *cotrimoxazole* 480 mg 1 tab x 2 / d for 3 days / week (watch for side-effects)

Lymphadeno-pathy	1. Adenopathy in a patient suffering from symptomatic HIV infection
	
	2. Chronic generalized lymphadenopathy = more than 3 lymph gland beds, at least 2 ganglions ≥ 1.5 cm / site, plus a month without other local or contignous cause of infection is generally due to AIDS infection
	
	Infection : *Neoplasia :*
	TB, Syphilis Kaposi's sarcoma
	Histoplasmosis Lymphoma
	Toxoplasmosis *Dermatological :*
	       Seborrheic
	HIV infection dermatitis
	       Chronic prodermitis
		1. Clinical
		Suspect TB or syphilis
		
		2. Suspicion of TB : needle biopsy of lymph mode + search for Koch's bacillus, X-Ray thorax
		
		3. Suspicion of syphilis
		Serology, direct examination
		
		4. If negative
		Biopsy is rarely indicated
			1. Tuberculosis
			Treatment see chap. 2
			Where TB is suspencte, give treatment on trial for 4 weeds, if improvment continues
			
			2. Syphilis
			Benzathine penicillin 2,4 MIU in a single dose
				Tuberculosis in a patient suffering from HIV infection is often extrapulmonary
				
				The diagnosis of chronic generalisized lymphadenopathy in an asymptomatic patient requires neither other investigations nor treatment
				
				The biopsy of a lymph mode may be indicated to exclude lymphoma, Kaposi's sarcoma or a fungal or mycobacterial infection

Table 22c

SYNDROME	DEFINITION AND ETIOLOGY	GUIDELINES FOR MANAGEMENT	TREATMENT
Cephalitis	The cephalitises in subjects suffering from symptomatic HIV infection are often persistent, severe, resistant to usual treatments *Infection :* TB meningitis Cryptococcal meningitis Meningo-encephalitic toxoplasmosis Neurosyphilis Viral meningo-encephalitis (CMV) Chronic HIV meningitis Multifocal leuco-encephalitis *Neoplasia :* Lymphoma Kaposi's sarcoma Common causes of encephalitis	1. Neurological evaluation : Altered psychol. state Focal attacks Convulsions Signs of meningism Intracranal hypertension 2. Look for malaria (if a fever) Thick and thin films 3. Lumbar puncture if no contraindication Diagnosis of TB, cryptococcus, bacterial meningitis	1. Where focal signs exist, treat for toxo-plasmosis for 6 weekss : ***pyrimethamine*** : loading dose 75-100 mg, then maintenance dose 25-50 mg/day + ***sulfadiazine*** 4-6 mg/day in 4 doses + ***folinic acid*** 15 mg/day 2. I thick-thin films are positive, treat for malaria (see chap. 5) 3. If lumpar puncture positive Bacterial meningitis : see chap. 7 TB meningitis : see chap. 2 Cryptococcal meningitis : ***amphotericine*** 0.4-0.6 mg/kg/d IV for 6 weeks or ***fluconazole*** 200-400 mg x 4/d orally-IV for 10 weeks 4. Cephalitis without recognisable etiology : symptomatic treatment beginning with simple analgesics	If treatment of toxo-plasmosis effective, long term prophylaxis is recommended : ***pyrimethamine*** 25 mg/day + ***sulfa-diazine*** 2-4 mg/day If cryptococcal meningitis, long term pro-phylaxis is necessary : ***fluconazole*** or ***ampho B***
Dermatological conditions	*Viral :* Herpes Herpes zoster Condyloma *Neoplasia :* Kaposi's sarcoma *Bacterial :* Furonculosis Impetigo Pyodermitis Hydradenitis Pyomyositis *Parasitic :* Chronic urticaria Seborrheic dermatosis Generalized erythroderma Psoriasis *Medication related* *Sexually transmitted diseases*		1. Viral infection Herpes zoster : local antiseptic treatment + ***acyclovir*** 800 mg x 5/d for 10 d + analgesics Herpes : see chap. 4 Condyloma : see chap. 9 2. Bacterial infection Furonculosis, impetigo, pyodermitis, folliculitis : local treatment + ***penicillin*** for 10 days Suppurative blisters : local treatment + ***tetracyclin*** 500 mg x 2/day for 6 weeks Pyomyositis : surgical drainage + antibiotics 3. Fungal infection Candidiasis : ***gentian violet*** or ***nystatin*** Fungal infections : see chap. 4

8

Prevention of transmission of HIV infection and AIDS

DURING SEXUAL INTERCOURSE

Systematic use of condoms is the only reliable prevention.

DURING TRANSFUSION

Strict respect for the indications for transfusion and systematic serological sampling of blood donors constitute the essential principals for the safety of transfusions.

See M.S.F. practical guide : *"Practical transfusion in isolated surroundings – prevention of transmission of HIV"*

IN MEDICAL FACILITIES

The prevention of the transmissin of HIV infection in the course of treatment takes place by reinforcement and strict respect for classical measures of hygiene :
– correct sterilization and disinfection of medical material,
– avoidance of injections which are not strictly necessary,
– precautions to avoid accidental contamination with soiled instruments,
– precautions to avoid contact with potentially infected biological liquids.

See M.S.F. practical guide : *"Recommendations to prevent HIV transmission in health care facilities in developing countries"*

Other conditions

9

Cardiac failure

☞ Syndrome characterized by the failure of the myocardium to maintain an adequate cardiac output. Often called congestive cardiac failure, or CCF.

Clinical features

– Exertional and paroxysmal nocturnal dyspnea (pulmonary edema).
– Hepatomegaly (tender liver on palpation).
– Ankle edema.
– Tachycardia with gallop rhythm.
– Basal crepitations on auscultation of both lung fields.

There are **3 forms** of cardiac failure :

– *Left ventricular failure*
  • Dyspnea : either exertional, recumbent (as in paroxysmal nocturnal dyspnea), or fulminant (acute pulmonary edema).
  • Crepitations (râles) in the lung bases on auscultation (may be absent in infants) ; sometimes pleural effusion.
  • Tachycardia, gallop rhythm.

– *Right ventricular failure*
  • Edema : especially of the ankles and lower legs.
  • large, tender, sometimes pulsatile liver.
  • Raised jugular venous pressure.

– *Biventricular failure* : combination of right and left sided signs.

Symptomatic treatment (hospital)

– Half-sitting position, oxygen if available.
– Exclude salt from diet.
– Drain any pleural effusion.

– Diuretics :

  • *Acute pulmonary edema*
    furosemide (IV)
    Adult : 20 to 40 mg/IV, repeated as needed
    Child : 1 mg/kg/IV, repeated as needed

9

- *Compensated cardiac failure*
  furosemide (PO)
  Adult : 20 mg/d divided in 2 doses
  Child : 1 to 2 mg/kg/d
  Furosemide therapy depletes potassium and therefore the patient should be supplemented :
  potassium chloride : 1 g/day, 5 days out of 7
  If furosemide is ineffective, use an aldosterone antagonist :
  spironolactone (PO)
  Adult : 100-200 mg/day in single dose
  Child : 3 mg/kg/day

- If furosemide or spironolactone are not immediately effective in acute pulmonary edema, two measures can reduce the load on the failing myocardium :
    - Rotating tourniquets : see pages 34-35.
    - Venesection : bleed 200 to 400 ml ; ensure first that significant anemia is not contributing to the cardiac failure.

- For left ventricular failure only

  - *In urgent situations* (e.g. acute failure)
    digoxin (IV)
    Adult : loading   : 0.25 mg/injection , 3-4 injections in first 24 hours
          maintenance : 0.25 mg/24 hours in 1 injection
    Child : loading   : 0.010 mg/kg/injection, 3-4 injections in first 24 hours
          maintenance : 0.010 mg/kg/24 hours in 1 injection

  - *In non urgent situations*
    digoxin (PO)
    Adult : loading   : 0.5 -1 mg/d divided in 2-3 doses x 2-3 days
          maintenance : 0.25 mg/d, for 5 days out of 7
    Child : loading   : 0.015 mg/kg/dose : 3-4 doses/24 hours x 2-3 days
          maintenance : 0.015 mg/kg/d in a single dose, for 5 days out of 7

- Treatment should be supervised : weight, dyspnea.

- Complications of treatment are bradycardia, arrhythmias and embolism.

- Pneumonia sometimes precipitates or complicates CCF. Treat with appropriate antibiotics (see pages 62-64).

Always seek a treatable cause.

The regimens below will usually be supplemented by symptomatic therapy of the CCF.

- *Anemia* : if severe enough to cause CCF may need transfusion (see page 29). Great care is needed because of the danger of fluid overload : usually **furosemide** is given at the same time as any transfusion.

- *Beri-beri* : think of this, especially in SE Asia
  thiamine (**vitamin B1**)
  Adult : 200 mg IM or IV/day
  Child : 50 to 100 mg IM or IV
  Continue with at least 200 mg/day PO for several weeks.

– *Endocarditis*
penicillin G (IV) : 100,000 IU/kg
+ **gentamicin** (IM) : 3 mg/kg/day

– *Chagas' disease* (see pages 135-136).

– *Acute rheumatic fever* : myocarditis may lead to CCF in the acute stage.
penicillin G or **PPF** (IM) : 100,000 IU/kg/d x 10 days.
prednisolone (PO) : 2 mg/kg/d x 3-5 days, then decreasing dose regimen over 7 to 10 days.

Prophylaxis :
benzathine penicillin (IM) : 1.2 - 2.4 MIU every 2 to 4 weeks.
< 15 years : 1.2 MIU every 2 weeks
> 15 years : 2.4 MIU every 2 weeks
for several months if possible.

9

Hypertension

☞ – Before diagnosing hypertension, the BP must be checked several times with *the subject resting*.

– *Drug therapy should only be instituted for BP consistently above 160/90 mmHg (or 140/90 for pregnant women).*

– Therapy must be *closely supervised*, otherwise side effects can be serious.

Treatment

ESSENTIAL HYPERTENSION *(dispensary)*

No evident cause, in a non-pregnant subject.

– Low-salt diet : follow-up one week later.

– If BP still > 160/90 : drug therapy.
hydrochlorthiazide (PO) : 50 mg/d, best taken in the morning.
Give *potassium* supplement (e.g. advise bananas in diet).

– If no improvement after one week give in addition :
methyldopa (PO) : commence with 250 mg/d divided in 2-3 doses, total dosage to be attended progressively 750 to 1,500 mg/d divided in 3 doses (upper limit).
or
hydralazine (PO) : 100 mg/d divided in 3-4 doses, if necessary can be increased till 200 mg/day

– Alternative :
propanolol (PO) : 40 mg/d (start with a low dose and increase slowly as needed. Do not let PR drop below 50-60/min).

HYPERTENSION OF PREGNANCY

Along with albuminuria and edema it is part of the syndrome of pre-eclampsia. This is a condition of late pregnancy and is associated with severe complications : eclampsia, abruptio placentæ and premature labour.

(dispensary)

– Rest, normal diet (do not restrict salt), encourage good protein intake.

– Sedation if necessary :
diazepam (PO) : 15 mg/d divided in 3 doses

- Observe regularly : BP, weight, albuminuria, edema, fetal heart sounds and movements, fundal height.

- If no improvement after one week :
  hydralazine (PO) : 100 mg/d divided in 3-4 doses (up to double this if needed)
  or
  methyldopa (PO) : 750 to 1500 mg/d divided in 3 doses

(hospital)

- Severe cases (very high BP, edema, headache, nausea, convulsions), i.e. preeclampsia :
  diazepam (IV) : 40 mg in 500 ml 5 % glucose infusion (to avoid risk of convulsions and lower BP).
  Definitive treatment : delivery, vaginal if possible.

- *Eclampsia*
  hydralazine (ampoule de 20 mg/ml, 1 ml) in infusion, protect from light, 4 ampoules of 20 mg in 500 ml 5 % glucose, delivered at 30 drops/minute, until normal BP achieved. Monitor rest of drip according to BP level.
  Convulsions : *diazepam* in infusion (see above).
  Nursing
  Obstetrical management : eventual caesarian.

9

Acute glomerulonephritis

☞ – An auto-immune inflammation of the renal tubules.

– Most often occurring as a complication of an otherwise benign streptococcal infection. Usually manifests itself 1 to 5 weeks following an episode of pharyngitis or impetigo.

– Affects mainly children over 3 years of age and adults.

Clinical features

– Proteinuria and hematuria.

– Hypertension, sometimes becoming malignant (encephalopathy).

– Edema.

– Occasionally cardiac failure.

Treatment *(dispensary - hospital)*

– Bed rest during the early period.

– Low salt diet.

– **Furosemide** (PO) if necessary : see above.

– Treat the hypertension (see pages 186-187).

– Treatment against the streptococci :
  • Acute phase : as for strep pharyngitis (see page 51)
  • Prophylaxis against relapse : as for rheumatic fever (see page 185)

Nephrotic syndrome

☞   – A syndrome that in its uncomplicated form comprises :
  - proteinuria (> 3 gram / 24 hours),
  - hypoalbuminemia (< 30 gram / litre),
  - edema.
  – These simple forms generally resolve completely. If complications are present (hematuria, hypertension, or renal failure), the disease has a poorer prognosis.

Treatment *(dispensary - hospital)*

– Rest.

– High protein diet.

– Restricted salt and water intake.

– Diuretics :
  furosemide (PO)
  Adult : 160 mg / d divided in 3-4 doses
  Child : 4 mg / kg / d divided in 3-4 doses
  Adapt dosage according to clinical response.

– For nephrotic syndrome in children, consider
  prednisone or *prednisolone* (PO) : 2 mg / kg / day x 5 days, then reduce dose progressively

9

Cystitis

☞   – Infection of the bladder and urethra, most often due to Escherichia coli.
      – Very frequent in women.

Clinical features

– Painful micturition (burning, scalding).

– Polyuria, nocturia.

– Urine cloudy and malodorous (sometimes hematuria).

– No fever.

Treatment *(dispensary)*

– Increase fluid intake : 3 to 4 litres/day, to flush out the bladder.

– Immediate antibiotic regimens (at the latest 3 days of beginning attack ; ensure no surgical operations or urinary infections during the last 3 months) :
  cotrimoxazole (PO) : 1.6 g of SMX in a single dose

– Standard antibiotic regimen :
  ampicillin (PO) : 2-3 g/d divided in 3 doses x 5-7 days
  or
  cotrimoxazole (PO) : 1.6 g of SMX/d divided in 2 doses x 3 days

– Exceptions
  • pregnant women :
    ampicillin (PO) : 2 g/d divided in 3 doses x 10 days
  • If signs of ascending infection (fever, chills, pain), treat as pyelonephritis (see page 192).

– Recurrent cystitis : think of schistosomiasis, urinary tuberculosis, a bladder stone or gonorrhoea.
  Otherwise, give antibiotic therapy for 10 days.

Lithiasis

 The formation of stones (calculi) in the urinary tract, which may cause varying degrees of obstruction.

Clinical features

- Renal colic : intense lumbar or pelvic pain, which may be either intermittent or constant.
- Hematuria, gravel in the urine, passing of a calculus.
- Microscopy : many red cells, sometimes some pus cells.
- Secondary infection is common : presents as cystitis or pyelonephritis.

Treatment *(dispensary)*

- Encourage copious oral fluids : at least 3 to 4 litres/day.
- Analgesia :
  noramidopyrine (PO) [1] : 1.5 g/d divided in 3 doses x 3 days
  + *butylhyoscine* (PO) : 30-60 mg/d divided in 3 doses x 3 days
- Antispasmodic :
  noramidopyrine (IV) [1] : 500 mg as required
  + *atropine* (IM) : 1 mg as required
- Secondary infections : treat appropriately.

[1] provided drug if prescribed in national list of the country.

9

Pyelonephritis

☞ Urinary tract infection involving the renal parenchyma, most often due to Escherichia coli.

Clinical features

- High fever (this may be the only sign in neonates).
- Chills, loin pain, dysuria, cloudy and sometimes bloody urine.
- Microscopy : abundant pus cells, red cells and bacteria on gram stain.

Treatment (dispensary - hospital)

- Treat the fever (see pages 26-27).

- Encourage abundant oral fluids (3 to 4 litres / day).

- *cotrimoxazole* (PO)
  Adult : 1.6 g of SMX/d divided in 2 doses x 10 days
  Child : 40 mg of SMX/kg/d divided in 2 doses x 10 days

- If very ill, or if cotrimoxazole ineffective after 3-4 days :
  ampicillin (IV) : 100 mg/kg/d divided in 4 injections for several days, then change to oral treatment (total : 10 days)
  + *gentamicin* (IM) : 3 mg/kg/d divided in 2-3 injections x 5-7 days

Prostatitis

 – Acute infection of the prostate gland.
– Usually due to gram negative bacteria.

Clinical features

– Scalding pain on urinating, polyuria, low grade fever and perineal pain.
– Tender on PR examination.
– Urine : pus cells, with occasionnal red cells.

Treatment *(dispensary)*

– Difficult to effect cure so often becomes a chronic infection.

– Encourage abundant oral fluids (3 to 4 litres/day).

– *cotrimoxazole* (PO) : 1.6 g of SMX/d divided in 2 doses x 2 weeks to 1 month.

– If this ineffective :
ampicillin (PO) : 2 g/d divided in 3 doses x 10 days

9

Sexually transmitted diseases (STD)

ATTENTION

All patients suffering from sexually transmitted disease are likely candidates for HIV (*i.e. practising non protected sexual intercourse*).

Urethritis

 Sexually transmitted infection of the urethra, most often gonococcal or chlamydial (the two may co-exist), occasional due to Trichomonas vaginalis or staphylococci.

Clinical features

– Incubation period 3 to 8 days.
– Often asymptomatic in females.
– Morning discharge from urethra with dysuria in males.
– Microscopic examination of fresh specimen of urethral discharge using gram stain (intracellular gram – diplococci). Always check partner(s).

Treatment (*dispensary*)

Whenever possible do a gram stain of the urethral discharge before starting treatment.

GONOCOCCUS (GRAM – DIPLOCOCCI ON GRAM STAIN)

– *cotrimoxazole* (PO) : 4 g of SMX/d in 1 dose x 3 days (= 10 tab 480 mg x 1 x 3 d)
– or *chloramphénicol* (PO) : 2.5 g/d in 1 dose x 2 days (= 10 tab 250 mg x 1 x 2 d)

of if available and recommended in regulations :
– *spectinomycine* IM : 2 g in a single dose
– or *kanamycine* IM : 2 g in a single dose

Then :
- *tetracycline* (PO) : 1.5-2 g/d divided in 3-4 doses x 7 days (except in pregnant or breast feeding women)
- or *doxycycline* (PO) : 200 mg/d divided in 2 doses x 7 days (except in pregnant or breast feeding women)
- or *erythromycin* (PO) : 1.5-2 g/d divided in 3-4 doses x 7 days

In region where gonococcal resistance is still rare :
- *PPF* IM : 4.8 MIU in a single dose (half given into each buttock)
- or *amoxicillin* (PO) : 3 g in a single dose

plus :
- *probenecid* (PO) : 1 g in a single dose
  probenecid is contraindicated in pregnant or breast feeding women.

then :
- *tetracycline*, or *doxycycline*, or *erythromycin* (see above).

TRICHOMONAS VAGINALIS

- *metronidazole* (PO) : 2 g in a single dose (= 8 tab 250 mg)
- or *metronidazole* (PO) : 750 mg/d divided in 3 doses x 7 days (= 1 tab 250 mg x 3 x 7 d)
  Metronidazole is contraindicated in the first trimester of pregnancy.

NO ORGANISM FOUND ON LABORATORY TESTING

Treat as a chlamydial infection :

- *tetracycline* (PO) : 1.5-2 g/d divided in 3-4 doses x 10 days

- or *doxycycline* (PO) : 200 mg/d divided in 2 doses x 10 days

- or, like for pregnant or breast feeding women :
  erythromycin (PO) : 1.5-2 g/d divided in 3-4 doses x 10 days

If no laboratory available, use one of the gonorrhoea treatment regimens above.

Always trace and treat all sexual contacts. Advise sexual abstinence or use barrier methods of contraception during treatment.

Evolution

If neglected, risk of re-infection and serious complications : prostatitis, salpingitis, pelvic peritonitis, septicaemia, arthritis and eventually infertility in females.

9

Syphilis

 A sexually transmitted disease due to Treponema pallidum.

Clinical features

Primary syphilis :
- Incubation period of 3 weeks (range 10 to 50 days).
- Single painless ulcer on the genitals with rounded, well-defined edge and indurated base. Sometimes there is inguinal adenopathy.
- Diagnosis often missed in women.
- Diagnosis by examining serous discharge from ulcer under dark-ground microscopy and by serology (VDRL, TPHA), Giemsa stain not advised because of other saprophyte treponemes in genito-perineal region.
- If untreated will evolve through secondary and tertiary stages.

Treatment (dispensary)

- **benzathine penicillin** : 2.4 MIU IM, repeated after 2 weeks.
- Trace and treat all sexual contacts.
- If allergic to penicillin:
  tetracycline or **erythromycin** (PO) : 2 g/d divided in 3-4 doses x 14 days

Prognosis

- If promptly treated, cure is complete.
- Untreated : evolution through secondary and tertiary stages.

Chancroid

 Sexually transmitted disease of which the causative agent is the Ducrey bacillus, Hæmophilus ducreyi.

Clinical features

- Incubation period of 3 to 5 days (range 1 to 15 days).
- Lone or multiple ulcers on the genitals (deep, painful, with a soft irregular base).
- Tender inguinal lymphadenopathy. Fistula formation may follow.
- Diagnosis is by smear from the ulcer (May-Grun-Wald-Giemsa stain).

Treatment (*dispensary*)

- *Cotrimoxazole* (PO) : 1.6 g of SMX/d divided in 2 doses x 10-15 days
  or *erythromycin* : 2 g/d divided in 3-4 doses x 10-15 days
- Trace and treat all sexual contacts.

Note : the ulcer may show sign of healing at the end of a week's treatment. If not suspect :
1. diagnostic error or tablets incorrectly or not taken ;
2. drug resistance ;
3. association with syphilis or AIDS.

Lymphogranuloma venereum

☞ A sexually transmitted disease, often abbreviated LGV, also known as Nicholas-Favre disease, and caused by Chlamydia trachomatis, especially in men, may be latent in women.

Clinical features

- Incubation period of 1 to 6 weeks.
- Small genital ulcer, not always present.
- Inguinal lymphadenopathy (nodes suppurate, ulcerate and communicate, forming fistulæ).

Treatment (*dispensary*)

- *tetracycline* (PO) : 1.5-2 g/d divided in 4 doses x 21 days
- Trace and treat all sexual contacts.
- Alternatives :
  • *erythromycin* : 1.5-2 g/d divided in 3-4 doses x 21 days
  • *cotrimoxazole* : 1.6 g of SMX/d divided in 2 doses x 21 days
- Never incise or drain lymph nodes as this retards healing. If necessary, aspirate fluctuant glands with a syringe through overlying healthy skin.

9

Donovanosis or granuloma inguinale

☞ Sexually transmitted disease also known as granuloma inguinale and due to Calymmatobacterium granulomatis. Much less common than LGV, it occurs in southern India, tropical and subtropical Africa, Papua New Guinea, South America and the Caribbean.
Non sexual contamination can occur (young children).

Clinical features

– Chronic painless granulomatous lesion of genitals.
– May also be inguinal or perineal.
– Develops over years if not treated.

Treatment (dispensary)

– Local disinfection.

– **tetracycline** (PO) : 2 g/d divided in 3-4 doses
or **ampicillin** (PO) : 2-3 g/d divided in 3-4 doses
or **cotrimoxazole** (PO) : 1600 mg of SMX/d divided in 2 doses
Therapy should continue until lesions healed (if not relapse occurs). Alternative therapy. Minimal course : 14 days.

– WHO recommends the systematic use of tetracycline with :
streptomycine IM : 1 g/d in single dose x 14 days
If this fails :
chloramphenicol (PO) : 1.5 g/d divided in 3 doses
+ **gentamicin** (IM) : 3 mg/kg/d divided in 3 doses
for 3 weeks

Genital herpes

☞ Sexually transmitted disease caused by herpes simplex virus.

Clinical features

– Multiple vesicles which evolve into tiny painful ulcers of the genitals.
– Attacks recur periodically.
– A benign condition except when it affects a pregnant women at delivery when there is a risk of disseminated infection in the neonate.

Treatment *(dispensary)*

– Reassure.

– Local disinfection with *chlorhexidine-cetrimide* solution or *chloramine* solution (preparation : see table 25, page 221).

– Apply *gentian violet* solution.

– Can relapse.

Condyloma acuminatum

☞ Raised wartlike lesions, found on the vulva or under the foreskin or on the skin of the anus.
Benign growth (papillomas).
Sexually transmitted viral infection.
Can deteriorate when atypical or pigmented conlyloma, biopsy.

Clinical picture

– Incubation period is several months.
– Single condylomatous lesion at beginning, which multiplies and grows and can become infected. Diagnosis is often missed in women.

Treatment

– Difficult to cure (frequent relapses).

– Previous local disinfection.

– Cautiously apply *podophylline* 10 or 20 % only to the growth. Leave it for 4 hours, then clean. Repeat every day for 3 to 4 days/week x 1.5 month <u>maximum</u>.

– Untimely and excessive treatment can cause painful ulcerations.

– *Podophylline* can be replaced by *trichloracetic acid* 80-90 % in same regime. Powder with talc or bicarbonate to remove excess acid.

– *Podophylline* and *trichloracetic acid* are contraindicated for cervical condylomas for which cryotherapy, electrocoagulation or surgical ablation should be used.

9

Vaginitis

 Infection of the vaginal mucosa caused by various pathogens : Candida albicans, Trichomonas vaginalis, Neisseria gonorrhœæ, Chlamydia trachomatis and others.

Clinical features

– White offensive vaginal discharge with itching, burning or discomfort.
– Diagnosis by direct smear (trichomoniasis, candidiasis) and gram stain (gonococcus).

Treatment (dispensary)

– *Candida albicans*
  • Douche with an alkaline solution :
  sodium bicarbonate or lemon juice or diluted vinegar (one teaspoon of vinegar in 1 liter of water).
  Or an antiseptic solution (*chlorhexidine-cetrimide*).
  • Apply *gentian violet* solution for 14 days.
  • Use *nystatin* vaginal pessaries : insert 1 each night x 10 days.

– *Trichomoniasis*
  • *metronidazole* (PO) : 2 g in single dose (gynaecological tablets are inefficient)
  • In case of failure, *metronidazole* (PO) : 1 g/d divided in 2 doses x 7 days

– *Gonorrhœa and chlamydia*
  Treat as for gonococcal urethritis, see page 194.

– *Non-specific vaginitis*
  • Douche several times daily with :
  chloramine solution diluted 1 in 2 (see table 25, page 221)
  or *povidone iodine* (10 % concentrated solution) diluted 1 in 20 for a few days
  • If no improvement after a few days :
  cotrimoxazole (PO) : 1.6 g of SMX/d divided in 2 doses x 7 days
  Pregnant women : *ampicillin* (PO) : 2 g/d divided in 3 doses x 7 days

– Treat all sexual partners.

Endometritis and Salpingitis

 A bacterial infection of the uterus (endometritis) or Fallopian tubes (salpingitis), sometimes causing pelvic peritonitis and septicemia. Often termed PID, the condition includes infections of both puerperal and venereal origins.

Clinical features

– Fever, abdominal pain, offensive discharge and sometimes bleeding.
– Vaginal exam : enlarged tender uterus.
– Speculum : pus emerging from the cervical os.
– Signs of peritonitis on abdominal palpation.

Etiological treatment

PUERPERAL SEPSIS *(hospital)*

Endometritis following delivery, miscarriage or abortion.

– **Post-partum sepsis** with no evident cause, retained placenta with secondary infection : usually streptococcal or gram negative.
  • **ampicillin** (IV) : 100 mg/kg/24 hours divided in 4 injections/24 hours
  • Observe progress closely, if no improvement :
    gentamicin (IM) : 3 mg/kg/24 hours divided in 3 injections/24 hours
  • Manual evacuation of the retained placenta. Wait until defervescence under antibiotics.

– Abortion (induced) (sometimes Clostridium perfringens).
  penicillin G (IV) : 100,000 IU/kg/24 hours divided in 4 injections x 10 days
  + **metronidazole** (PO) : 1.5 g/d divided in 3 doses x10 days.

VENEREAL INFECTIONS *(hospital)*

– Same clinical picture as above, or else an isolated salpingitis, either gonococcal or chlamydial.

– Laboratory confirmation is preferable.

– Give IV antibiotics :
  Penicillin G (IV) : 100,000 IU/kg/24 hours divided in 4 injections/24 hours x 3 to 5 days, then continue with once daily **PPF** (or **procain penicilline**)
  or
  ampicillin (IV) : 100 mg/kg divided in 4 injections/24 hours

9

– For chlamydia :
tetracycline (PO) : 2 g/d divided in 3 doses x 10 days.
or
erythromycin (PO) : 50 mg/d divided in 3 doses x 10 day

– If in doubt, give :

penicillin G or **ampicillin**	with	**tetracycline** or **erythromycin**

IN CASES OF PUERPERAL SEPSIS AND VENEREAL INFECTION WITH NO BACTERIAL CONFIRMATION

– In the absence of bacteriological confirmation and if there are signs of peritonitis, give :
    ampicillin (IV) : 100 mg/kg/24 hours divided in 3 injections x at least 10 days
+ **gentamicin** (IM) : 3 mg/kg/24 hours divided in 2 injections x 8 days
+ **metronidazole** (PO) : 1.5 g/d divided in 3 doses x 10 days

– At the end of the treatment, continue with :
tetracycline (PO) : 1.5 g/d divided in 3 doses x 10 days

– In cases of an abscess in the pouch of Douglas, pyosalpinx or diffuse peritonitis, *hospitalize for surgical treatment.*

PV bleeding

☞ – Vaginal bleeding other than during menstruation. The origin may be vaginal, cervical or uterine.

– If chronic, anemia may occur.

– If hemorrhage is profuse, shock is likely. Nurse patient supine, observe pulse and BP, establish IV line, check hematocrit and restore blood volume.

Bleeding in the non-pregnant patient

PRE-PUBERTAL GIRLS *(dispensary)*

– Eliminate :
  • trauma or foreign body,
  • vaginal tumour (rare).
– Treat appropriately : remove foreign body and suture traumatic wounds.

WOMEN OF CHILDBEARING AGE *(dispensary)*

Diagnosis depends on clinical examination of the vagina with/without speculum.

– Cervicitis or ectropion : inflamed cervix, sometimes associated with vaginitis. Exclude cervical cancer, take a smear for bacteriological diagnosis and treat as for vaginitis.

– Cervical cancer : surgery if available.

– Normal cervix with enlarged uterus : exclude pregnancy (see following page).

– If uterine fibroids :
  norethisterone (PO) : 5 to 10 mg/day from the 10th till the 25th day of the menstrual cycle for 3 cycles, then adapt according to response.
  Surgery if no improvement.

– Normal cervix, normal uterus with adnexial mass : exclude ectopic pregnancy. Chronic : ovarian cyst, hydrosalpinx. Surgical referral.

9

- Normal examination :
  - With an oral contraceptive or *Depo-Provera bleeding can be due to poor compliance or poor tolerance.
  - Uterine polyp.
  - Functional menorrhagia or endometrial hypertrophy, consider :
    norethisterone (PO) : 5 to 10 mg/day from the 10th till the 25th day of the menstrual (PO) : 5-10 mg/day from day 15-25 of menstrual cycle
  - Schistosomiasis : check for eggs of S. hæmatobium in the urine (see page 114).

MENOPAUSAL WOMEN

- Endometrial carcinoma (uterus sometimes enlarged). Hysterectomy if surgical facilities available.

N.B. :
In all of the above situations anemia must be prevented or corrected with :
ferrous sulphate + *folic acid* (PO) : 6 tab/d divided in 3 doses x 1-2 months.

Bleeding during pregnancy

FIRST TRIMESTER *(hospital)*

Miscarriage (spontaneous abortion) : contractions and bleeding.

- Establish IV line, restore volume if shocked, observe pulse and BP.
- 3 stages :
  - Cervix closed (threatened miscarriage). Bed rest, monitor vital signs.
  - Cervix open, sometimes with expulsion of products (inevitable abortion). If does not progress, curettage may be necessary (digital after 2 months gestation).
  - Uterus involuted, products expelled (completed abortion). Curettage if suspicion of retained products of conception.
- Antibiotic prophylaxis :
  PPF (or *procain penicillin*) (IM) : 4 MIU/d x at least 5 days.

Induced abortion (patient may deny it)

- Manage as for miscarriage plus broad-spectrum antibiotic cover :
  ampicillin (IV) : 100 mg/kg/d divided in 4 injections x 7 days
  or
  chloramphenicol (IV) : 75 mg/kg/d divided in 4 injections x 7 days.
- If a clostridium perfringens infection is suspected, treat with :
  penicillin G (IV) : 100,000 IU/kg//24 hours divided in 4 injections x 10 days
  + *metronidazole* (PO) : 1500 mg/d divided in 3 doses x 10 days

Ectopic pregnancy : bleeding, pelvic pain, malaise and shock.

- The uterus is of normal size or a little enlarged.
- PV exam : marked adnexial tenderness and in pouch of Douglas.
- There is a danger of rupture leading to hemoperitoneum, exsanguination and death.
- IV line, resuscitation, transfusion as needed.
- Urgent laparotomy.

Hydatidiform mole (relatively common in North Africa and Asia)

- Shortly after conception there is bleeding and often severe nausea and vomiting, and the uterus is larger than expected.
- Grape-like vesicles may be expelled.
- IV line, suction or digital curettage (not instrumental, as danger of perforation).
- Prolonged follow-up because of risk of choriocarcinome : pregnancy tests or HCG levels if available, initially every fortnight, then monthly for at least a year. Provide effective contraception during this period.

Third trimester

(hospital)

Premature labour : scanty bleeding, contractions before term, cervix may be open and effaced, uterus non-tender, examination otherwise normal

- Bed rest.
- *salbutamol* infusion : 3 mg (6 amp of 0.5 mg/ml) in glucose or normal saline over 24 hours. Monitor the rate of infusion, pulse and BP, and fœtal heart rate.
- Continue therapy for 24 hours after the contractions cease.

(hospital)

Placenta prævia : profuse painless hemorrhage

- Patient supine, establish IV line. Monitor pulse, BP, blood loss and fœtal heart rate. Transfusion as needed (consider HIV).
- If in premature labour, treat accordingly (see above).
- If full term and in labour and partial placenta prævia only, rupture membranes and attempt vaginal delivery.
- If bleeding intractable, or if complete placenta prævia, deliver by cæsarian section.

9

Abruptio placentæ : also known as accidental hemorrhage or retro-placental hematoma.

It is caused by premature separation of a normally inserted placenta. Frequent antecedents are pre-eclampsia or trauma (road accident or a beating). Bleeding may only be minimally evident vaginally and the amount seen bears little relation to actual blood loss. There is severe continuous abdominal pain, shock and a hard uterus. The fetus is often dead. Disseminated intravascular coagulation may occur as a complication.

− Establish IV line, transfuse to maintain stable vital signs.

− Live fetus perform a cæsarian section.

− If vital signs are stable and labour is advanced or there is a dead fetus, vaginal delivery should be attempted.
Rupture membranes.
Give analgesia :
pentazocine (IM) : 30 mg
+ *butylhyoscine* (IV) as needed.
Induction and augmentation :
oxytocin : 5 IU in 500 ml 5% glucose, adapt rate of infusion in terms of response.
Forceps or vacuum extraction may be necessary.
Beware of post-partum hemorrhage.

(hospital)

Post-partum hemorrhage (PPH)

− After all deliveries the pulse, BP and blood loss should be monitored. Normal loss is less than 500 ml.

− If there is PPH (> 500 ml).

− Establish IV line. Restore blood volume as necessary with plasma volume expanders or whole blood (see page 29).

− Careful examination to determine cause of hemorrhage :
  • Retained placental tissue.
  • Uterine atony : if uterus not contracted, exclude retained placenta (requires manual removal).
  • Lacerations : perineum, vagina, cervix (inspect the cervix by drawing it gently forward with the help of a scrubbed assistant using three sponge forceps).
  • Coagulopathy.

− Treatment :
  • Manual exploration of the uterine cavity whenever there is the slightest doubt (anesthesia, full aseptic technique) followed by :
  methylergometrine : 0.2 mg IV thence IM 2 or 3 times/day
  + *ampicillin* prophylaxis.

- Suture any bleeding lacerations.
- Replace blood losses by transfusion where available. If coagulopathy is suspected, transfuse with fresh blood.
- Follow-up with *ferrous sulphate* + *folic acid* for 2 months.

Late PPH : subacute bleeding accompanied by fever is probably due to a retained placenta with secondary infection.

– Treat appropriately (see page 201).

9

Toothache : different syndromes

 Toothache is a common complaint. The causes are multiple but there are seven identifiable syndromes :

– Pain induced by cold (rather than heat), by acidic foods, by sugar, and relieved once the stimulus is removed, is caused by *dental caries.*

– Pain spontaneous, intermittent and radiating, is caused by a nerve exposed by *advanced caries.*

– Pain induced by cold, heat, acidic foods, sugar and persisting for several minutes after suppression of the stimulus is due to *pulpitis.*

– Pain which is spontaneous, continuous, intense, throbbing, exacerbated by heat and percussion on the affected tooth, not relieved by ordinary analgesics, is caused by a *dentoalveolar (periapical) abscess.*

– Congestive or suppurative pericoronitis, with pain, redness, and swelling of the gum, and sometimes pus, is caused by the *eruption of teeth* (e.g. wisdom teeth).

– Shooting pains exacerbated by movements of the tongue and swallowing, with localized swelling, are due to a *suppurative cellulitis.*

– Pains of variable intensity associated with bleeding gums are due to *gingivitis*, irritation or scurvy.

Treatment (dispensary)

All patients should receive scaling and simple instructions on dental hygiene. Specific therapy (see table 23, page 209).

Table 23 : *Dental conditions and treatment*

Clinical Forms	Conservative treatment	Extraction	Analgesic	Antibiotic	Anti-inflammatory
Dental caies	If possible		±		
Exposed nerve and pulpitis	If possible	Immediate			
Dentoalveolar (periapical), abscess	If possible	Immediate or after 24 h of antibiotic	*Paracetamol* per os Ad. : 2 g/d divided in 4 doses Ch. : 30 to 50 mg /kg/d divided in 4 dosess Avoid acetylsalycilic acid in case extraction becomes necessary	*Ampicillin* per os Ad. : 2 g/d divided in 3 doses for 6 days Ch. : 50 to 100 mg/kg/d divided in 3 doses for 6 days	*Indomethacin* per os Ad. : 75 mg/d divided in 3 doses x 3 days Ch. 3 years and + (15 kg) : 37.5 mg/d divided in 3 doses Ch. 5 years (20 kg) 50 mg/d divided in 3 doses Ch. 10 years and + (30 kg) : same as adult
Malaligned erupting teeth		After 24 hours of antibiotic if infected			
Localized cellulitis		After 24 hours of antibiotic			
Gingivitis	Treat the cause (scurvy ?)			If infected	If infected

9

Dental infections

 Infection arising as a complication of inflammation of the dental pulp.

There are three main syndromes.

LOCALIZED INFECTIONS

Dentoalveolar or periapical abscess.

– *Acute* : intense continuous throbbing pain, looseness of the affected tooth with expression of pus.
– *Chronic* : apical granuloma, sometimes with cyst formation. May be asymptomatic (incidental X-ray diagnosis) or be tender to percussion. May become reinfected.

CIRCUMSCRIBED INFECTIONS

Less localized than a periapical abscess.

– *Acute serous cellulitis* : swollen gum around tooth, pulsatile, mobile, with no fluctuation.
– *Acute suppurative cellulitis* : fever, malaise, gum swollen and very tender, with fluctuation.
– *Acute gangrenous cellulitis* : as with suppuration, plus crepitations on palpation.
– *Chronic cellulitis* : burnt out but may become secondarily infected. Marked by a painless nodule.

DIFFUSE INFECTIONS

Cellulitis that spreads through the adjacent facial and cervical tissues. May lead to necrosis and septicemia.

Dental infections may metastasize to distant sites. Think of a dental focus in cases of bacterial endocarditis, prolonged PUO, or abscess of organs.

Treatment *(dispensary)*

Table 24 : *Dental infections and treatment*

	Root canal therapy (dentist)	Extraction	Incision and drainage	Antibiotic	Anti-inflammatory
Acute peri-apical abscess	If possible	Immediate	No	***Ampicillin*** per os	***Indomethacin*** per os
Chronic peri-apical abscess	If possible	Immediate	No	Adult : 2 g/d divided in 3 doses for 5 days	Adult : 75 mg/d divided in 3 doses for 3 days
Cellulitis	If possible without antibiotic	24 hours after of A.B. treatment	No	Child : 50 to 100 mg/ kg/d divided in 3 doses for 5 days	Child : 3 years and + : 37.5 mg/d divided in 3 doses
Cellulitis with abscess	If possible without antibiotic	24 hours after of A.B. treatment	24 hours after of A.B. treatment		> 5 years (20 kg) : 50 mg/d divided in 3 doses > 10 years (30 kg) : as adult x 3 days
Gangrenous cellulitis	No	24 hours after of A.B. treatment	24 hours after of A.B. treatment with lavage using A.B.	As for diffuse cellulitis (below)	
Diffuse cellulitis	No	Infusion IV (***glucose*** 5 %) ***ampicillin*** IV 4 x 1 g Supervision ++ If necessary : ***gentamicin*** IM 3 mg/kg divided in 2 IM/d x 5 to 7 days As soon as possible, ***ampicillin*** IM or per os			

9

Endemic goitre

 Goitre is a swelling of the neck due to enlargement of the thyroid gland.
This may be due to problems of thyroid function (genetic deficit, hypophyso-hypothalamic control desorders) or a tumor.
However, the main cause of goiter in tropical countries is dietary iodine deficiency. Moreover, some food contains goitergenic factors : manioc and cruciferous (cabbage...).
Goitre is an adaptive process. The deficit in thyroid hormone synthesis due to iodine lack is compensated by a hypertrophy of the gland. Most cases of goiter are euthyroid.

Clinical features

The WHO proposes a classification according to the type of enlargement. The different grades of this classification are as follows :

- *Group 0* : thyroid is non palpable or palpable, but volume of the lobes is smaller than the distal phalange of the patient's thumb.

- *Group 1a* : thyroid is easily palpable. The volume of the lobes is larger than the distal phalange of the patient's thumb.

- *Group 1b* : as above, thyroid is visible in an extended neck, but not in normal position.

- *Group 2* : thyroid easily visible when the head is in normal position.

- *Group 3* : thyroid enlargement visible at a distance of 5 meters.

Meantime, one could also classify goiter according to its diffuse, nodular or multinodular characteristics.

Complications

- *Locally* : swallowing disorders, collateral circulation, tracheal compression, severe respiratory disorders, sudden enlargements especially during puberty and pregnancy. Rarely cancerous.

- *Complications of subclinical hypothyroidism in pregnancy include* : Low birth weight, congenital malformations and high perinatal mortality. Fetus, newborn and infant can present with hypothyroidism (cretinism with mental retardation neurological disorders and retarded psychomotor development).

Treatment

Goitre is an adaptation to a chronic lack of iodine.
Surgery should not be considered except in cases with severe complications (rare).

Prevention

The aim is to reduce the complications in new borns and infants. Prevention in the long term would have an impact on the rate of goiter in the population. There are 3 methods :

– *Iodising cooking salt with iodure or potassium iodate*
This technique is used in several countries and its effectiveness has been proved, but it requires a large program at national level.

– *Intramusculary iodine oil injection*
It has been shown that 1 ml iodine oil injections ($\pm$ 0.48 g iode) in adults and 0.5 ml in children make goiters regress. It normalizes the thyroid function and prevents cretinism in the new-born for a period of 3 to 5 years.
For this treatment to have an impact on the community, a global program is necessary. It should not be used for individual treatment as it is relatively expensive.

– *Oral iodine solution (Lugol®)*
Adult : 2 ml PO
Child < 1 year : 1 ml PO
This treatment is covering needs for 1 to 2 years.

9

CHAPTER 10

Medical and minor surgical procedures

10

Dressings

☞ Dressing is a set of procedures for treating a wound. A wound is an interuption in the continuity of the skin secondary to trauma or surgery.

Objectives

– *Protection*
  • To prevent contamination from the external environment.
  • To protect against possible trauma.

– *Cicatrisation*
  To favour tissue regeneration.

– *Absorption*
  To absorb serous discharge.

– *Disinfection*
  To destroy pathogenic organisms.

– *Compression*
  To stop hemorrhage.

Warning : a dressing occludes a wound and in certain conditions (humidity, heat) can encourage multiplication of pathogenic organisms.

Equipment

– 1 box of sterile instruments
  • 1 set of dissection forceps
  • 1 set of Kocher forceps
  • 1 pair of scissors
– 1 dressing tray (clean)
– 1 drum of sterile gauze pads
– 1 kidney dish
– Cotton wool (for equipment disinfection only, never use cotton wool directly on a wound)
– Adhesive tape
– Flasks containing antiseptics :
  chloramine and / or *chlorhexidine-cetrimide*, and *polyvidone iodine* (dilution : see table 25, page 221).
  N.B. : Never use polyvidone iodine with soaps containing mercurial derivatives.
  Solution preparation should be rigorous. Solutions should be renewed every week (every 3 days for chloramine).

10

General rules of asepsis

– A room should be kept for dressings. It should be carefully cleaned everyday and dressing tables should be disinfected between each patient.

– Use a sterile box of instruments for each dressing, or at least for each patient.

– Always start from the clean area and move to the dirty one.

– Wash hands carefully after each dressing, and after removing bandages or adhesive tape.

Technique

EQUIPMENT AND INSTRUMENT PREPARATION

– Cleaning of the dressing tray with *chlorhexidine-cetrimide*.

REMOVAL OF THE PREVIOUS DRESSING

– Removal of bandages and adhesive tape (not the gauze pads).

– Hand washing (clean water + soap).

– Removal of gauze pads, using Kocher forceps
  • If the dressing adheres, soak it with sodium chloride solution or an antiseptic.
  • Act gently not to remove the granulating epidermis.

WOUND EXAMINATION

– **Sutured wound and/or aseptic wound**
  • Check the stage of cicatrization if wound is weeping, has a hematoma, or is infected.

– **Septic wound**
  • Check the nature of secretions and if there are new fleshy pimples.
  • A bluish pus indicates the presence of pyocianic (quickly spreading, very resistant bacillus spreading very quickly).
  • Look for any signs of lymphangitis.
  • Use new forceps after removal of the dirty dressing and the first cleaning of the wound.

CLEANING OF THE WOUND

– Use the sterile dissection forceps to remove sterile gauze pads from the container, and place them on the tray.

– To make a sterile sponge fold the pads twice using the Kocher and dissection forceps (as illustrated).

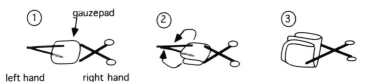

① gauzepad ② ③

left hand   right hand

– Pour an antiseptic solution on the pad (infected wound, burns, abcess, ulcers: *chlorhexidine-cetrimide* ; non infected surgical wound : *polyvidone iodine* ; see table 25, page 221).

– Clean the periphery of the wound either with a circular movement, or from top to bottom. Change gauze pads as often as necessary.

– Clean the wound from top to bottom with a new tampon.

– Dry the periphery of the wound and then the wound itself with different gauze pads.

DRESSING A WOUND

– Apply one or several gauze pads to the wound.

– Apply strips of adhesive tape :
  • perpendicularly to the axis of the limb or the body ;
  • Leave the central part free to avoid maceration.

N.B. : When sterile disposable material is limited, sterile pads should be reserved for aseptic and surgical wounds.

Frequency of dressings

– *Surgical wounds, or non infected sutures*
  • First day dressing should be well protected.
  • Further dressings, every 48 to 72 h (check the process of recovery).

– *Infected wounds*
  • Dress every 24 h.

– *Deep or large burns*
  • Dress on the first day, then leave until the 7th day (unless obvious infection).

– *Phagedenic ulcers*
  • Dress every 24 h, with hospitalisation if possible.

10

Associated antibiotic treatment

As a rule, systemic antibiotic treatment should not be prescribed routinely.

– *Deep and soiled wounds,* to prevent gas gangrene
procain-penicillin (IM) : 4 or 5 IU per day x 5 days at least.

– *Abcess*
Antibiotic treatment is useless before incision.

– *Burns*
Only if they are infected.

– *During conflicts or other disaster relief conditions,* where access to health care and patient's follow-up are hazardous, the systematic use of *PPF* (or *procain-penicillin*) should be considered.

Wastes

All soiled disposable materials (gauze, coton, dressings, etc...) should be collected and burned daily.

Choice and use of antiseptics and disinfectants

See table 25, following page.

Table 25 : *Antiseptic and disinfectant*

INDICATIONS	PRODUCT TO USE	DILUTION	STORAGE	REMARKS
– *Fresh wounds* – *Washing hands* (e.g. before injections) – *Cleaning skin* – *Perineal cleaning before delivery*	CHLORHEXIDINE (1.5 %) + CETRIMIDE (15 %) = HAC® or Savlon® or CHLORHEXIDINE (5 %) or ORDINARY SOAP	20 ml per 1 litre 10 ml per 1 litre Use water from the water mains (running water) or water filtered by a candle type filter and boiled for 5mn.	Renew once a week	Never use for wounds to the skull or ear. Never use with soap.
– *Infected wounds* (pus, smell…) – *Abscess* – *Furuncles* – *Infected ulcers…* (anything purulent)	TOSYLCHLORAMIDE SODIUM	5 g per litre (2 g per litre for mucosa or when used frequently) (equivalent to DAKIN solution) Rinse the bottle abundantly before each preparation.	Renew once a week	Put in a brown or opaque bottle (non metal containers). In case of prolonged use, protect the healthy skin around the wound with vaseline
– *Mycoses* (e.g. thrush) – *Running dermatoses* (eczema, impetigo) – *Superficial burns* – *Small and superficial wounds*	GENTIAN VIOLET	Saturated solution (5 g/l) 1 teaspoon/litre Shake several times, leave for some time and pour into another bottle or filter to remove any deposit.	Renew once a week	Do not use on the face of light skinned people, as it can provoke persistant pigmentation.
– *Placement of IV catheter,* *lumbar puncture* – *Umbilical cord* – *Surgical procedure* – *Surgical wounds before suture*	POLYVIDONE IODINE (10 %) = PVI	Pure (= 10 % PVI)		
– *Post-operative care* (change of dressing) – *Site of injection*	= Betadine®	2.5 % PVI : 1 part of 10 % solution + 3 parts of filtered and boiled water.	Renew once a week	Never use with a mercury derivative (Merfen®, Mercurochrome®, disinfectant liquid soap).
– *Floors, mattresses,* *tables, kidney-dishes,* *drawsheets…*	LYSOL or chlorinated SOLUTION	Lysol : 20 to 50 ml/litre depending on the amount of dirt. Bleach 12° (4 % chlorine) : 50 ml/litre Calcium hypochlorite (70 % chlorine) : 3 g/litre (2 tablespoons per 10 litres of water) Chloramine : 5 g/litre	Prepare just before use	Precautions for the use of chlorinated solutions : do not use a metal container and do not mix with a detergent. Clean dirty surfaces before application.

10

Abscess

 A collection of pus in the soft tissues. An abscess cavity is not accessible to antibiotics.
Treatment is thus surgical only.

Indications

Incision and drainage (I & D) should be performed once the abscess is "ripe" i.e. fluctuant upon gentle palpation.

Material

- Sterile scalpel blade and handle.
- Surgical gloves.
- Plain curved forceps (Kelly forceps).
- Sterile corrugated drain.
- Antiseptic solution e.g. *chloramine* solution or *chlorhexidine-cetrimide* solution (preparation : see table 25, page 221).
- 5 or 10 ml syringe.

Anesthesia

Anesthesia of an abscess by local infiltration with *lidocaine* is not very effective. Furthermore, the act of traversing wider areas of tissue with a needle may spread the infection further. Regional anesthesia is preferable where possible : e.g. ring block of a finger. Otherwise, the skin can be briefly numbed using *ethyl chloride* spray.
General anesthesia may be necessary for an abscess that is large or deep such as some breast abscesses, "injection" abscesses of the buttock, and pyomyositis : *ketamine* 1-2 mg/kg by slow IV or 5-10 mg/kg IM. The smaller IV dose acts more rapidly and for a shorter time than an IM dose and may thus be preferable.

Technique

- Scalpel : the correct way to hold a scalpel is between the thumb and forefinger with the handle resting against the palm (see Figure 7a). It should not be held as one holds a pen. The plane of the scalpel blade should be perpendicular to the plane of the skin.
- Incision : the free hand immobilizes the wall of the abscess between thumb and forefinger. Incise in the long axis of the abscess with a single stroke to breach the skin. The incision should be long enough to allow insertion of an exploring finger.
- Precautions : take care not to incise too deeply if the abscess overlies major blood vessels (the carotid, axillary, humeral, femoral and popliteal regions). After breaching the skin, blunt dissect down to the cavity using Kelly's forceps.

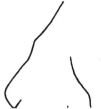

Figure 7a
Position of the hands for incision of an abscess

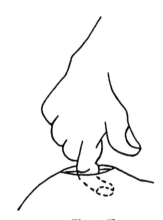

Figure 7b
Exploration of the cavity with a finger in order to break down loculations

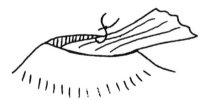

Figure 7c
Drain fixed to the skin

Figures 7 : *Technique for incision and drainage of an abscess*

- Explore the cavity with the forefinger, breaking any loculating adhesions and evacuating the pus (see Figure 7b).
- Abundant lavage of the cavity using a syringe filled with *chloramine* solution or *chlorhexidine-cetrimide* solution (preparation : see table 25, page 221).
- Insert a drain, if possible fixing it with a single suture at the edge of the incision. The drain is withdrawn progressively then removed altogether after 3 to 5 days (see Figure 7c).

10

BREAST ABSCESS

(see Figures 8a to 8d)

– The management of breast abscess is slightly different. Usually the abscess is superficial but deep ones, when they occur, are more difficult to diagnose and to treat.
– Early in the infection, before the infection loculates (mastitis), non-surgical measures should be applied :
  • Antibiotics :
    ampicillin (PO) : 100 mg/kg/d x 5 days
    or
    chloramphenicol (PO) : 75 mg/kg/d x 5 days.
  • Anti-inflammatories :
    indomethacin (PO) : 75 mg/d divided in 3 doses x 3 days
  • Hot compresses, a constricting bandage to reduce lactation in the affected breast and expression of milk to avoid engorgement.

Material
– Same material as for other abscesses (see above).

Technique
– Incision :
  • for superficial abscess : radial
  • for abscess near nipple : peri-alveolar
  • for deep abcess : beneath the breast
– Gentle exploration with finger or Kelly forceps.
– Abundant lavage with *chloramine* solution or *chlorhexidine-cetrimide* solution.
– Insertion of drain.

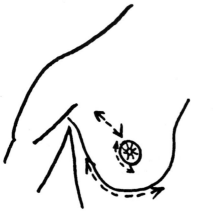

Figure 8a
Incisions : radial, peri-areolar
or submammary

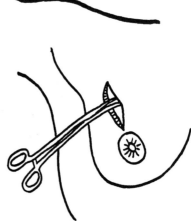

Figure 8b
Exploration (gentle) with a finger
of forceps

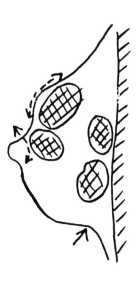

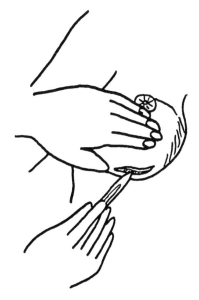

Figure 8c
Common sites for breast abscess

Figure 8d
Submammary incision

ABSCESS IN THE PAROTID REGION

There is a danger of sectioning the branches of the facial nerve. The incision should be over the caudal part of the abscess and parallel to the lower border of the maxilla (see Figure 9).

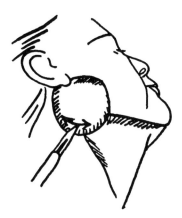

Figure 9 : *Horizontal incision for parotid abscess*

10

Pyomyositis

☞ Infection and eventually abscess formation within muscle, most often due to Staphylococcus aureus.

At the start of infection, when the muscle is swollen, hot and painful, medical treatment may *prevent abscess formation : immobilize, give antiinflammatory medication* (*indomethacin* (PO) : 75 mg/d divided in 3 doses x 5 days) and antibiotics (*ampicillin* (PO) : Adult : 4 g/d in divided 3 doses ; Child : 100 mg/kg/d divided in 3 doses x 7 days).

Indication

If the swelling becomes fluctuant conduct an exploratory puncture with a large-bore needle which will reveal thick pus.

Material

The same that for an abscess.

Anesthesia

Use *ketamine* (IM) if needed (see page 222).

Technique for abscess drainage

– Generous skin incision, avoiding underlying neurovascular tracts, and incision of the fascia and muscle sheath, also with the scalpel (see Figure 10a).

– Blunt dissection with Kelly forceps down to the abcess cavity (see Figure 10b).

– Exploration with a finger to break adhesions and evacuate the pus (see Figure 10c).

– Abundant lavage with *chloramine* solution or *chlorhexidine-cetrimide* solution.

– Where possible, counter-incision of the skin near the edge of the abcess, cutting down onto a finger that is inserted deep in the cavity. The counter-incision should be anatomically posterior to the abscess to allow gravity drainage (assuming the patient will be supine during recovery). A strip of corrugated drain is threaded through the two incisions (see Figure 10d), fixed with a suture to the edge of the incision and withdrawn around the 5th day.

Note : Myositis of the right psoas muscle may present in a manner identical to that of acute appendicitis. Surgical evacuation is necessary.

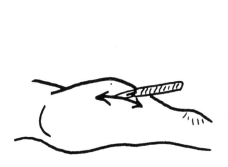

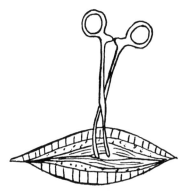

Figure 10a
Generous incision

Figure 10b
Blunt dissection of muscle using
Kelly forceps : insert closed then
withdraw slightly opened

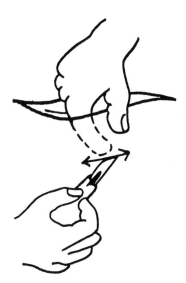

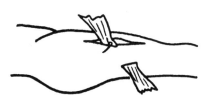

Figure 10c
Counter-incision for drain, cutting down
into finger inserted deep in cavity

Figure 10d
Drain passing through
the two incisions

Figures 10 : *Technique for incision of muscle abscess*

10

Burns

☞ | Thermal trauma to the skin, mucosa and deeper tissues. Burns are classified according to depth and extent.
Any burn that affects greater than 10 % of the body surface area is considered extensive and is thus serious because of fluid loss, cata-bolism, anemia and the risk of secondary infection. Burns are very common in rural societies, particularly among children who fall onto or roll into cooking fires.

Clinical features

The extent of a burn is expressed as a percentage of total body surface area involved, easily estimated by the "rule of nines" (Table 26). The degree is a function of the depth to which tissue damage penetrates (Table 27).

A patient with extensive burns is likely to be in shock and requires appropriate resuscitation. Among children, the younger the patient the graver the danger presented by a burn of given extent and degree.

Table 26 : *"Rule of nines" for calculating percentage of body surface burned*

Body area	Adult (%)	Child (%)
Entire head	9	18
Upper limb	9	9
Anterior or posterior surface of trunk	18	18
Lower limb	18	14
Perineum	1	1

Table 27 : *Depth of burns*

1st degree	Skin red and tender
2nd degree superficial	Skin red with blistering, tender to touch
2nd degree deep	Skin white, dry and soft Diminished sensibility to touch or pin-prick
3rd degree	Black skin, diminished sensibility to touch or pin-prick

Treatment

FIRST AID

– Immerse in cold water ; this provides good analgesia and also arrests on-going trauma due to the heat retained in the tissues.
– Apply *gentian violet.*
– Do not cover.

RESUSCITATION

– Calculate the fluid requirements for the first 24 hours : weight x % of surface burn x 2 = quantity of fluid required in mls.
  e.g. : 60 kg (wt) x 20 % (extent of burn)
          60 x 20 x 2 = 2,400 ml
– 75 % of fluid should be given or *ringer's lactate*, the remainder as volume expanders or blood transfusion.
– During the first 24 hours, half the fluid requirements should be given in the first 8 hours.

FIRST DRESSING OF THE BURN

– Analgesia (*pentazocine* IM : 30 mg) and sedation if necessary (*diazepam* IM : 10 mg).
– Tetanus prophylaxis if available.
– Strict aseptic technique : drapes, gloves and instruments all sterile (Figure 11).
– Clean the burn with normal saline or *chlorhexidine-cetrimide* solution (see table 25, page 221).
– Use a scalpel to debride blisters and non-viable tissue.
– Apply sterile vaseline gauze, then on top of that two layers of unfolded sterile gauze swabs. Do not use either antibiotic ointment or gauze impregnated with antibiotics or corticosteroids.
– Apply a bandage, *not tightly.* Do not wrap limbs, especially at the flexures as this will encourage contractures. *Bandage each finger separately*, never together.
– Immobilize limbs in the position of function.
– Alternatively : "open method" : after wound cleaning *leave the burn uncovered with the patient protected by a mosquito net.*

SUBSEQUENT DRESSINGS

– Unless infection ensues, the first dressing should be left undisturbed for 5 to 7 days.
– Analgesia aseptic technique as for the first dressing.
– Remove any black eschars (which may hide purulent areas) and use scalpel to excise any necrotic tissue : skin, aponeurosis, muscle or tendon.

10

– Systemic antibiotics if obvious infection (not antibiotic ointment) :
  PPF (or **procain penicillin**) (IM) :
  Adult : 4 MIU/d x 5 days at least
  Child : 100,000 IU/kg/d x 5 days at least
– Same dressing as the first time. Again, this should not be removed for 5 to 7 days.
  Healing is signaled by granulation tissue : pink, mat and clean.

PATCH GRAFTING

(Figure 12)
– Skin grafting is necessary when the wound is slow to heal : often the case with
  deep second degree and third degree burns. Patch grafting is a simple technique
  and can also be used for treating tropical ulcers once the base is clean and
  granulating.
– Aseptic technique. Shave the donor area (usually anterior thigh or forearm) and
  prep with **povidone iodine** (see table 25, page 221). Infiltrate with **lidocaine** 1%.
– Lift up a patch of skin with fine toothed forceps and excise it with a scalpel. It
  should be full-thickness i.e. epidermis plus dermis. Take other patches from
  different parts of the donor site, leaving areas of intact skin between each excision.
– Spread each patch out on a sterile swab dampened with normal saline.
– Once a sufficient number of patches are excised, apply them carefully to the
  wound. Do not place them too close together : further healing will bridge the gaps
  and this allows a larger area to be grafted.
– Dress the donor and graft sites with sterile vaseline gauze, then layers of swabs
  and a non-compressive bandage.
– The graft will take within 7 days, during which time the dressing should not be
  removed and the patient should remain as immobile as possible.

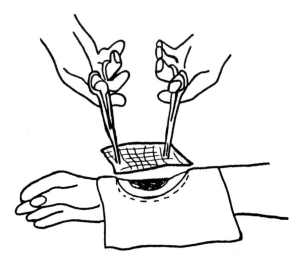

Figure 11
Dressing a burn : sterile technique, use of vaseline-gauze

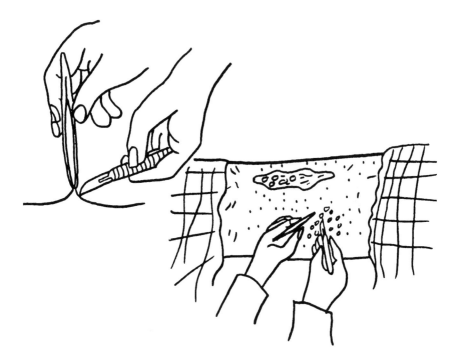

Figure 12
Full-thickness patch skin graft :
sterile technique, taking of donor patches using a fine toothed-forceps and a scalpel

Wounds

General principles

This chapter concerns only wounds that can be treated at a dispensary level. For major trauma, refer to a surgical manual.

- Immediate ("primary") closure of wounds is desirable but not always practi-cable and in some circumstances it may be dangerous (risk of infection).
- Classically, it is said that a wound of greater than 6 hours should not be sutured. In isolated rural practice, however, patients often present late because of distances and this limit may be extended up to 24 hours, provided the patient can be observed during the following days for signs of infection.
- An infected wound should never be sutured.
- *War wounds, animal and human bites should not be sutured.*
- Any break in the skin overlying a fracture is an "open fracture".
- A wound that communicates with a joint is an open joint wound.
- Always give antitetanus prophylaxis if available.

The following are steps in the treatment of a wound : preparation, explo-ration, debridement, closure, drainage, and finally removal of sutures.

Preparation

WOUND TOILET

Shave if necessary, then clean the wound and its periphery with *polyvidone iodine* (see table 25, page 221).

MATERIAL

(Figures 13a to 13c and 14a to 14d)
- Sterile gloves and fenestrated drapes.
- *Lidocaine*, needle and syringe.
- Suture material.
- Suture set (sterilized box of instruments) : needle holder, needles, scalpel blade and handle, one or two artery forceps, fine curved scissors with rounded ends, plain scissors for cutting sutures, retractors.

LOCAL ANESTHESIA

- Only necessary for large or deep wounds requiring more than 2 stitches.
- *Lidocaine* 1% without adrenaline.
- Infiltrate subcutaneously via the wound edges.

Exploration

Once anesthetized, the wound can be explored and thoroughly cleaned of any debris. Have a gloved assistant using retractors if necessary. Be careful to exclude the following :
– Foreign body.
– Underlying fracture.
– Involvement of nerves, major blood vessels, tendons or joints.
– For scalp wounds : underlying fracture (if serious may contain brain tissue).

Closure

– Use interrupted sutures (not continuous).
– Non-resorbable sutures such as silk for skin, resorbable thread (chromic catgut, Vicryl®...) for subcutaneous tissues.
– Some suture material is already mounted on a needle by the manufacturer ("atraumatic needles").
– A curved needle is easier to manipulate.
– For skin use a "cutting" needle (triangular in cross-section) ; for subcutaneous tissues use a "round" needle (circular in cross-section).

Table 28 : *Suture materials recommended for different wounds*

Skin of face	Nylon (no resorbable)	dec. 2.5 (= 3/0*)
Skin of scalp	Nylon (no resorbable)	dec. 3 (= 2/0)
Skin of limbs or trunk	Nylon (no resorbable)	dec. 2.5 or 3 (= 3/0 or 2/0)
Subcutaneous tissue	Resorbable synthetic**	dec. 3 (= 2/0)
Aponeurosis	Resorbable synthetic	dec. 3 (= 2/0)
Muscle	Resorbable synthetic	dec. 3 (= 2/0)

* From 0 to 3/0 the suture becomes increasingly fine in caliber.
** Resorbable synthetic : resorbs slowly (over 3 weeks), e.g. vicryl®...

Drainage

– Use a strip of corrugated rubber drain.
– Never use a drain for wounds of the face.
– Always insert a drain in wounds of the scalp and whenever a hematoma can be expected to form.

Removal of sutures

Face : day 5 ; other wounds : day 7 or 8.

10

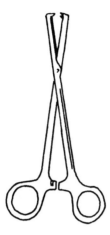

Figure 13a
Kocher forceps
toothed

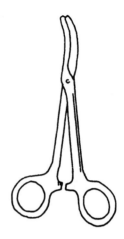

Figure 13b
Kelly clamp
curved, untoothed

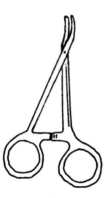

Figure 13c
Mosquito forceps curved and untoothed
(also called artery clamp or hemostat)

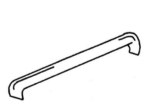

Figure 13d
Retractor (Farabeuf type)

Figures 13 : *Different instruments*

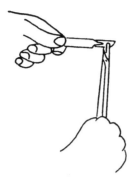

Figure 14a
Always mount a scalpel blande using a needle holder.
Change blades for each different operation (even on the same patient).

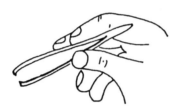

Figure 14b
Dissecting (toothed) forceps should not be held in the palm
but between the thumb and index finger. They should be used on skin only.

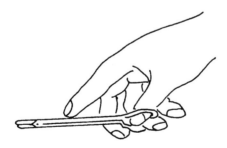

Figure 14c
Insert the thumb and the ring finger into the handle of a needle holder (or scissors),
and stabilize the instrument using the index finger.

Figures 14 : *How to hold instruments*

10

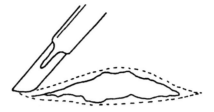

Figure 15a
Debridement of a contused, messy wound : straightening of wound edges
with a scalpel. Be very careful on the face.

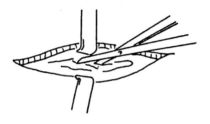

Figure 15b
Excision of torn edges of aponeurosis to avoid necrosis.

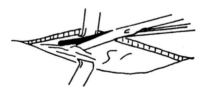

Figure 15c
Excision of torn or contused muscle.

Figures 15 : *Debridement*
(this should be sparing, limited to excision of severely contused or lacerated tissue
that is evidently destined for necrosis.)

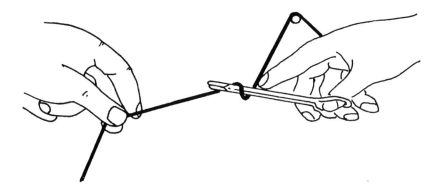

Figure 16a
Loop the suture material around the needle-holder in one direction (e.g. "over towards me") and remember this direction.
Take the loose end with the needle holder and pull it throuth to make the first knot.

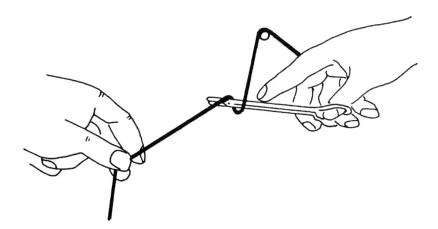

Figure 16b
The second loop should be in the opposite direction ("under towards me").
Repeat a third knot, changing direction once again.

Figures 16 : *Practice with knots*

10

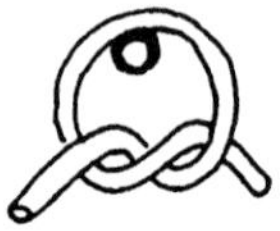

Figure 16c
The first knot should be flat.

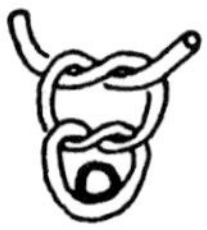

Figure 16d
Second knot : opposite direction.

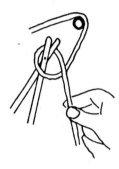

Figure 16e 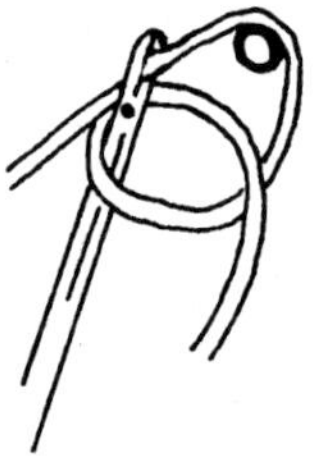   **Figure 16f**
Catching the loose end with the needle-holder.

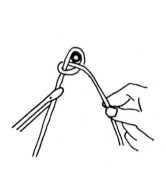

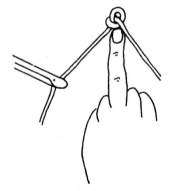

Figure 16g   **Figure 16h**
Slip the knot up towards the nail using the hand that holds the free end,
holding the other length of suture with the needle-holder.

Figures 16 : *Practice with knots* (continued)

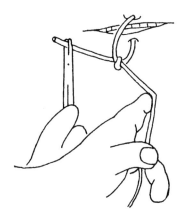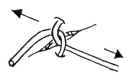

Figure 17a
First knot flat

Figure 17b
Tighten without causing ischemia (pallor)

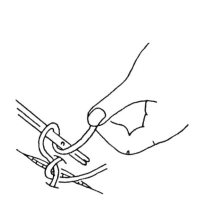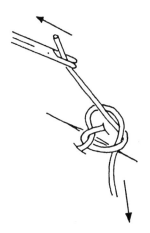

Figure 17a
Loose end pulled through

Figure 17b
Second knot in opposite direction

Figures 17 : *Tying knots on skin*

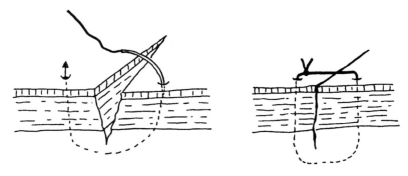

Figure 18a   **Figure 18b**
The "bite" taken must be sufficiently deep.

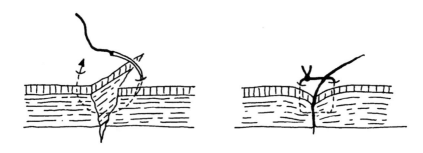

Figure 18c   **Figure 18d**
Incorrect : bite too shallow, so the edges invaginate.

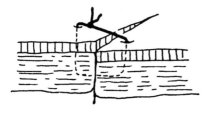 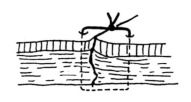

Figure 18e   **Figure 18f**
Incorrect : poor opposition of the edges   Incorrect : the knot should be beside
the wound, not over it.

Figures 18 : *Particular problems*

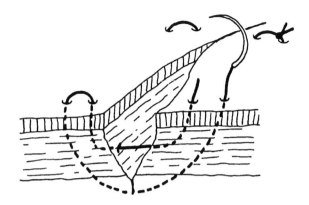

Figure 19 : *Vertical mattress suture (also called Blair-Donati technique)* : allows good apposition of the wound edges.

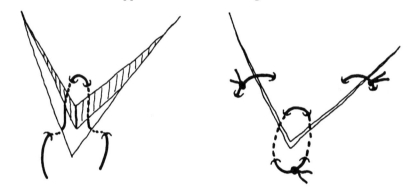

Figure 20 : *Closing a corner*

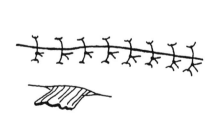

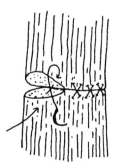

Figure 21
Close skin using interrupted silk or nylon.
In case of deep wound, a drain is usually advisable (emerging via a counterincision) to avoid hematoma.

Figure 22
Repair of muscle using interrupted sutures throuth the full thickness. Use chromic (or Vicryl...) crossed in X.

10

Bites and stings

☞ Trauma caused by venomous animals ; bites are inflicted by the mouth-parts (e.g. snakes, spiders), stings by the hindparts (e.g. bees, scorpions).

Treatment (*hospital*)

ENVENOMATION BY INSECTS, SCORPIONS AND SPIDERS

– *Stings by bees, wasps...*
Usually benign, but in susceptible individuals may provoke either laryngeal edema or anaphylactic shock :
adrenaline (*epinephrine*) (SC) :
Adult : 1 mg
Child : 0.01 mg/kg
dexamethasone (IV) : 4 mg stat. Repeat if required
plus a perfusion of *ringer's lactate* or volume expander.

– *Spider bites and scorpion stings*
Gravity depends upon the particular species, however the majority of such envenomations are either benign or else cause local tissue damage only. If a truly toxic species is thought to be responsible apply first aid and supportive measures as for snakebite (see below). Otherwise, therapy is limited to analgesia, local wound toilet and reassurance.
Clean and disinfect wound :
noramidopyrine (IM) (or any other analgesic) : 500 mg in 1 injection IM
If pain very severe :
pentazocine (IM) : 30 mg in injection IM
or *lidocaine* 1% (without adrenaline) infiltrated around the wound gives good relief for very painful scorpion stings.

SNAKEBITE

It is most often not possible to identify the snake reponsible. In any case, the principles of management are the same : first aid and supportive therapy as indicated from close monitoring of the victim's clinical condition. Antivenenes are costly, difficult to store, difficult to use, sometimes dangerous (anaphylaxis), and moreover of arguable efficacy.
– *First aid* : the "pressure-immobilization method". The object is to confine the venom to the site of the bite, thus allowing time for the body to metabolize it and for attendants to transport the victim to a health care facility. Venom diffuses mainly via the lymphatics, not via blood, tourniquets are thus of little use.
  • Apply firm constant pressure to the site of the bite.
  • Apply a crêpe bandage (or substitute) firmly to the entire limb.
  • Immobilize the limb with a splint.
  • Immobilize the patient.
– *Supportive therapy* : see table, following page.

Table 29 : *Snake-bite*

Time since bite	Clinical pictures	Treatment
5 minutes	Bite visible Pain	First aid (see text)
15 minutes	Anxiety Numbness Nausea Dyspnea	Establish IV line Antitetanus prophylaxis Observation
30 minutes to 3 hours	Shock	Rapid IV infusion (plasma volume expanders if available)
	Paralysis Respiratory failure	Endotracheal intubation Manual ventilation
	Haemorrhagic syndrom Shock (due to hemolysis and disseminated intravascular coagulation)	Transfusion of fresh blood
	Edema Local inflammation	***PPF*** (or ***procaïne pénicilline***) Adult : 4 MIU/d IM Child : 100,000 IU/kg/d for at least 5 days ***Dexamethasone*** IV or IM : 6 to 12 mg/d for 3 days
More than 3 hours	No symptoms	Reassurance, home
	Necrosis	Daily dressings Continue ***PPF*** Debride, graft as needed Amputation if needed

10

Appendix

Disinfection and Sterilization of medical equipment and supplies

☞ – *Sterilization* = elimination of all micro-organisms (viruses, microscopic fungi, bacteria, both vegetative and spore forms).

– *Disinfection* = elimination of most micro-organisms present on a surface or object.

– *Decontamination* = disinfection of object soiled by infectious material (pus, blood, excreta...).

General rules

All equipment or supplies :
– coming into contact with sterile parts of the body (injection equipment, surgical instruments, some dressings, catheters...).
– used for perfusion.
should be sterilized and kept sterile until utilization.

All reusable items, which do not correspond to the above definition, but which come into contact with mucus membranes, or get soiled with pus, blood, lymphatic or vaginal secretions, should be sterilized or subjected to a *high level disinfection* (effective among others against HIV and hepatitis B virus).

All soiled, non reusable equipment *should be incinerated* (warning : never recap needles after use = main cause of accidental needlestick).

To carry out proper sterilization is not always easy in the field conditions of isolated rural medical centers. It requires proper appliances (autoclave, hot air sterilizer), and an energy source.
In practice, one is often obliged to use alternative procedures which are not wholly satisfactory as they produce disinfection rather than sterilization (They are however compulsory if one cannot do better) (see following chapters).

Disinfection and sterilization of medical equipment is not enough to prevent iatrogenic infections (resulting from medical practice). It is obvious that basic hygienic and asepsis techniques ought to be applied : cleaning and disinfection of surfaces and premises, personal hygiene of the staff, aseptic handling of sterilized instruments...

247

Cleaning of reusable equipment

Soiled items and instruments should be carefully cleaned before being sterilized or subjected to a final disinfection.

The presence of organic matter could protect germs against the action of a disinfectant or sterilizing agent, or could react against it, rendering it ineffective.

INSTRUMENTS

Cleaning can be done either with water alone, with water and soap (or detergent), or with water and a compound of disinfectant/detergent.

Cleaning with a disinfectant chemical aims mainly to reduce the risks of contamination for the staff, but it does not eliminate them completely.

The staff in charge of instrument cleaning should be aware of the contamination risks (AIDS, hepatitis B), they should wear thick plastic or rubber gloves, and be careful when they handle sharp instruments.

After use and before cleaning, all instruments and items should be soaked in water to avoid deposits drying up. A disinfectant could be added for a first decontamination (chloramine 20 g/l, lysol 50 g/l).

Metallic instruments can be damaged if they are left in water too long (over several hours) or if the disinfectant concentration is too high.

Note

Needles and syringes for immunization should be soaked and cleaned with water alone, as traces of soap and disinfectant can inactivate vaccines.

After cleaning, instruments and items should be rinsed thoroughly with water and dried, then sterilized, boiled or disinfected (with a high level disinfectant) depending on their use and the local sterilizing facilities.

LINEN AND DRESSING

To decontaminate linen and dressings, one should wash them with an ordinary washing powder (eg. OMO) and boil them if possible (5 minutes).

If boiling is not possible, linen should be washed, rinsed and soaked for 30 minutes, in a 0.1 % chlorine solution (hypochlorite, bleach, chloramine), or 5 % lysol solution. It should then be rinsed abundantly and dried.

Theatre linen should be sterilized in an autoclave or ironed depending on local facilities.

Sterilization methods and alternatives

AUTOCLAVING

Sterilisation by steam under pressure in an autoclave.

Autoclaving is the most reliable sterilization method and the only one that allows effective sterilization of all medical equipment and supplies (especially linen and rubber). But relatively sophisticated appliances and energy source (electricity, kerosene or gas) are needed.

It is based on the same principle as a kitchen pressure cooker. Because water is heated in a closed container, temperatures above 100°C can be reached.

In the absence of air (air is purged at the beginning of sterilization), the temperature can be regulated by controlling the pressure.

According to the type of supply to be sterilized, sterilisation is carried out at 121°C (1 atmosphere over atmospheric pressure) or at 134°C (2 atm. over atmospheric pressure).

Items to be sterilized	Temperature		Pressure*		Duration **
	°C	°F	Atm., Bar or kg/cm^2	PSI	
Instruments, syringes, plastic, glass, rubber	121	250	1	15	30'
Dressing (swabs), linen (gowns, drapes...)	134	275	2	30	20'
	Otherwise 121	250	1	15	40'

* Over atmospheric pressure
** Add 5 minutes per 1000 meters above sea level

Note :

– Do not forget to expell air (purge) while increasing the pressure (otherwise the temperature in the autoclave will not be sufficient).

– Drums or boxes holding objects to be sterilized must be open, never closed (unless fenestrated). The sliding windows in the special autoclave boxes should also be open during sterilization.

– Count the sterilizing time from the moment the required temperature or pressure is reached, not from the start of the heating phase.

Dry heat (in hot air sterilizer or oven - called a Poupinel in french)

Sterilization by hot air (dry heat) at 160°C (320°F) for 2 hours or at 170°C (340°F) for 1 hour.

Reliable method provided it is carried out in a good electric appliance with working thermometer (an air circulation device is needed in large ovens).

This method is convenient for metal, heat resistant glass, and vaseline, but is not convenient for linen or gauze swabs. The oven method is quite simple but consumes more energy than an autoclave.

Ovens heated by charcoal fires or kerosene heaters are not reliable because they do not produce a sufficiently high temperature.

Time should be calculated from the moment the required temperature is reached (this is very important).

Notes

- Begin heating with the door open to expel any humidity (which could rust instruments).
- Do not exceed 170°C (could damage metallic instruments).
- It is better to place items in closed boxes. However, large boxes should be left half-open to allow the material to more rapidly achieve the correct temperature.

Boiling

Boiling for 20 min (adding 5 minutes for 1000 altitude) provides high level disinfection, but not sterilization because it does not destroy bacterial spores (eg. : tetanus, gangrene).

Boiling is nevertheless essential when autoclaving or hot air sterilization are not possible. It is particulary useful for needles and syringes (it destroys HIV and hepatitis B virus).

After needles and syringes have been boiled, they should be kept dry and not left in the water (which can easily become recontaminated).

Flaming

- *In a flame* : Effective if instruments are made red hot. This method should only be used in exceptional circumstances as it damages metal.
- *With alcohol* : Instruments are dipped in alcohol and set alight. This method is unreliable, expensive and in the long term damages instruments.

Ironing

Surgical drapes and gauzes can be ironed if an autoclave is either unavailable or too small to hold large operating drapes.

Iron on a table or bench covered with a sheet that has itself just been "sterilized" by ironing.

Dampen each item slightly with filtered boiled water.

The iron should be very hot and passed several times over each side of the linen/gauze.

However, if it is available, autoclaving is always the preferred method.

Immersion (of *clean* equipment) in the following disinfectant solutions destroys bacteria and virus including HIV and hepatitis B virus. The bacterial spores are generally not destroyed.
This process could be used as an alternative to sterilization when autoclaving or hot air sterilization are not possible.
Boiling however is always preferred. The effectiveness of chemical disinfection can always be impaired by dilution errors, by bad storage conditions, or by prolonged utilization of the same solution (solutions should be renewed at least once a day).
Chemical disinfection should never be recommended for syringes and needles.

	Recommended concentration	Preparation	Minimal contact	Note See below
Hypochlorites	0.1 % of active chlorine (1,000 ppm)	see note 1	15 min.	**2**
Tosylchloramide Chloramine T	2 %	20 g/litre	15 min.	**3**
Polyvidone iodine (Povidone iodine, PVI)	2,5 %	1 part 10 % concentrated solution + 3 parts water	15 min.	**3**
Ethanol	70 %	8 parts ethanol 90 % + 2 parts water	15 min.	**4**
Isopropanol	70 %	7 parts isopropanol + 3 parts water	15 min.	**4**
Formaldehyde	4 %	1 part formalin + 3 parts water	30 min.	**5**
Glutaraldehyde	2 %	Addition of the activator supplied with the solution	30 min.	**5**

1. Hypochlorite solution (0.1 % or 1,000 ppm[1] available chlorine) is prepared either from liquid bleach recently manufactured (< 3 months) or from calcium hypochlorite or from sodium dichloroisocyanurate (NaDCC, "Javel tablets", Javel solid®, Stafilex®, Actisan®...), diluted according their respective available chlorine content.
Fresh liquid bleaches contain 3 to 15 % available chlorine (sometimes expressed in chlorometric degrees, 1° chlorom. = approx. 0.3 % available chlorine). Calcium hypochlorite contents from 30 to 70 % available chlorine. The NaDCC based tablets content generally 1.5 g available chlorine per tablet (1 tablet per litre = 1,500 ppm available chlorine).

NaDCC withstands heat much better than bleach and calcium hypochlorite.

---

[1] 1 ppm = 1 part per million = 1 mg/l

2. As hypochlorite solutions are corrosive for metal, these solutions are convenient only for good quality stainless steel. The soaking should not exceed 1/2 hour and should be followed by thorough rinsing.

3. If instruments are used immediatly after soaking, it is not necessary to rinse the chloramine or the polyvidone iodine solution.

4. Ethanol and isopropylic alcohol (isopropanol) should be used at 70 % (70°) for the best effectiveness (more concentrated solutions are less effective). The prices, transportation and importation problems limit the use of these alcohols.

5. Immersion for several hours in aldehyde solutions, formaldehyde (formalin) and glutaraldehyde (Cidex®), provides proper sterilization (destruction of all germs). These solutions however have many disadvantages : thorough rinsing compulsory (toxic residues), toxic vapours (formalin), high cost (glutaraldehyde).

Notes

– In order to obtain effective disinfection, *equipment must be cleaned before immersion in all these solutions...*

– Aqueous solutions of cetrimide (Cetavlon®), chlorhexidine (Hibitane®), Savlon®, HAC®, Dettol® and other common detergent and disinfectant solutions do not provide sufficient disinfection.
Soaking instruments in these solutions with the aim of "sterilization" should be avoided. This only provides an illusive feeling of safety and could in fact be a source of contamination.

STERILIZING GASES

– *Ethylene oxide*
This method cannot be considered in field conditions because of its cost and of the special installation it requires (ethylene oxide is very toxic).

– *Formol vapour* (paraformaldehyde or trioxymethylene or "formol" tablets and Aldhylene®)
Formol autoclaving also cannot be considered in the field. However formol vapour is often used for "makeshift" sterilization of instruments. The instruments are thoroughly cleaned and dried, then placed in a airtight container for at least 24 hours (minimum temperature of 20°C), either along with formol tablets 5 tablets for 1 litre container) , or with formol alcoholic solution (Aldhylene®) (1 ml for 1 litre container). Afterwards instruments are rinsed with sterile water. This is often impracticable, but it is absolutely compulsory if there is any visible deposit.
Users should be cautious during manipulation as vapors are toxic and highly irritative.
This method is not suitable for linen or gauze swabs as they absorb formaldehyde, which is toxic and necroses skin and mucus membranes.
This method is not totally reliable and has many disadvantages. It should be abandoned. If it is used an effective disinfection method against HIV (AIDS virus) (eg. boiling) should always be carried out before hand.

Equipment and methods recommended

DISPENSARIES

Recommended equipment
- 1 small autoclave pressure cooker type (volume 15 to 20 litres)
- 1 powerful kerosene stove (or electric hot-plate)
- 1 metal mesh basket
- Appropriate fenestrated containers (drums)

Recommended methods
- Instruments, syringes, glass, rubber, plastic, gauze swabs, small drapes : autoclave.
- Large drapes, gowns : wash with soap powder, boil if possible, then "sterilize" by ironing.

MOBILE TEAMS

Recommended equipment
If possible same equipment as for dispensaries.
Otherwise :
- 1 container for boiling
- Chloramine T or Polyvidone iodine (Bétadine®)

Recommended methods
As for dispensaries if possible.
Otherwise :
- Metal instruments : boiling (best), otherwise sodium dichloroisocyanurate (NaDCC) or chloramine T or polyvidone iodine (exceptionally, after boiling and drying, instruments may be kept with formol tablet or Aldhylene® until utilization)
- Needles, syringes : boiling
- Swabs : use disposable supplies

HOSPITALS WITH SURGICAL FACILITIES

Recommended equipment
Same equipment as for dispensaries and :
- 1 large autoclave (interior dimensions about 40 x 60 cm), operating with electricity, gas or kerosene according to local conditions.
- 2 mesh baskets
- Several fenestrated drums (number according to activity)
- Several fenestrated instrument boxes
If electric current is available continuously for at least 3 hours per day :
- 1 electric hot air sterilizer

Recommended methods
- Metal instruments, glass : hot air sterilizer if good electric apparatus available, other-wise autoclave
- Swabs, linen (gowns, drapes...) : large autoclave
- Rubber, plastic items, syringes : small or large autoclave (at 121°)

Directions for use of an autolcave

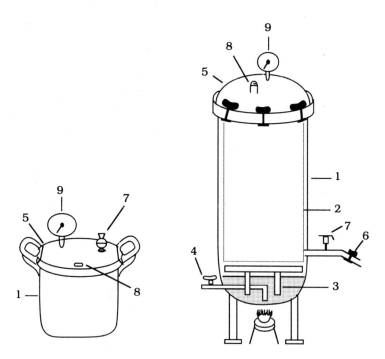

1. Body of the autoclave

2. Mesh basket to contain packages to be sterilized

3. Metal base to support basket, drums above water

4. Drain tap

5. Lid, usually with a rubber seal and bolt-type catches

6. Tap or valve to allow purging of air during heating phase

7. Pressure valve : regulates the pressure by allowing excess vapour to escape

8. Safety valve

9. Pressure gauge

Note

In small autoclave, pressure cooker type, there is no purging tape, one uses the valve for purging.

The safety valve should not be manipulated during autoclaving (it will function only in case of excessive pressure rise).

Pressure gauge shows a pressure scale and sometimes a temperature scale.

Pressure could be indicated in different manners.

One may consider that 1 bar = 1 kg/cm^2 = 1 atmosphere = 15 psi

Temperature could be indicated in °C ou °F (135°C = 275°F ; 121°C = 250°F).

OPERATION

1. Put the require quantity of water in the autoclave before each sterilization (dry heating could damage the autoclave) : the level is usually marked or the quantity indicated by the manufacturer. If possible use distilled water or filtered rain water.

2. Place the objects to be sterilized in the mesh basket or onto the support, leaving enough room for vapour to circulate freely. The sliding "windows" on drums or containers must be open. Do not overload the autoclave.

3. Close the lid by tightening the bolds in diametrically opposite pairs (as the wheel nuts of a vehicle).

4. With the purging tap or valve open, begin to heat.

5. When a continuous jet of vapour is coming out of this tap/valve, close it.

6. Allow the pressure to rise to 0.5 atm, then open the purge tap/valve for 10 seconds to purge air, then close it.

7. Repeat this purge at about 0.7 atm, then again at about 0.9 atm.After this, all air should have been expelled from the autoclave and only steam will remain.

8. When desired operating pressure (and thus temperature) is obtained, sterilization begins. Start to time it then, not before.
   The pressure valve regulates the pressure inside the autoclave allowing excess steam escape. There may be two interchangeable valves or positions to operate at either 1 or 2 atm.. If a lot of steam is being expelled, heat source should be lowered slightly.

9. After the required duration of sterilization, shut off the heat source.

10. Evacuate water and steam :
    – For large autoclaves : through drain tap (to be connected outside).
    – For pressure cooker type autoclaves : evacuate the steam by opening the purge valve. Once pressure drops to zero, open the lid, lift out the basket, pour out the water then replace the basket.

11. Allow to cool with the lid slightly open. Residual heat helps dry the sterilized items (the danger of contamination by ambiant air is minimal).

12. Once items are dry, close the sliding windows on drums.

Note

If the autoclave is equiped with a drying system, follow the manufacturer's recommendations starting from paragraph 9.

PRESSURE OR TEMPERATURE AND DURATION REQUIREMENTS

Items to be sterilized	Temperature		Pressure*		Duration **
	°C	°F	Atm., Bar or kg/cm²	PSI	
Instruments, syringes, plastic, glass, rubber	121	250	1	15	30'
Dressing (swabs), linen (gowns, drapes...)	134	275	2	30	20'
	Otherwise 121	250	1	15	40'

* Over atmospheric pressure
** Add 5 minutes per 1000 meters above sea level

OPERATION VERIFICATION

- The stove should be powerfull enough to obtain a minimum rise of pressure of 1 atmosphere (1 bar or 1 kg/cm² or 15 Psi).
- If possible, use sterilization autoclave tests, for example, 3M Autoclave Tape should turn black, brown is insufficient).
  Warning, do not confuse test tape for hot air sterilizers with that for autoclaves.They are very similar but not interchangeable.
  Place tests (eg. strip of tape) in the middle of the load into the boxes or drums to ensure that sterilization (temperature, steam, duration) is completed.

PACKAGING OF ITEMS FOR STERILIZATION

- Packaging of items : either
  • without package if items are to be used immediatly,
  • fenestrated drums or boxes,
  • heavy duty paper : wrapping paper, kraft paper or news paper (2 layers),
  • closely-woven linen (2 layers),
  • mixed (1 layer of paper, 1 layer of linen).
  Paper plus linen is advisable if item is to be stored several weeks (because more resistant than paper alone and best barrier for germs than linen alone).

- Fenestrated containers should be equiped with a filter (a layer of heavy duty paper see above) accross the windows within the container or around the load to be sterilized so as to filter air during the drying phase after auto-claving. The paper should be checked and renewed regularly.

- If the autoclave is not equiped with a drying system, drying up of items inside boxes and drums is often unsastifactory. It is easier when the items are packed with paper or linen.

- Packed items should be placed vertically in the autoclave basket (not lying flat).

- Small packages and small drums are preferable to large ones.

- Needles and syringes : separate plunger and barrel of syringes and stick needles onto a gauze swab.

- Swabs and drapes should not be compressed inside boxes or drums.

Monthly epidemiological report

The goal of this report is to facilitate and standardize data collection for epidemiological surveys. It should record the monthly activities of the program and help in constructing the three-month and yearly reports. This form is a frame work for data collection, it should be adapted to the specific program.

Identification

Country   : ....   Month : ....

Place or site : ....   Year   : ....

Population

MONTHLY REPORT

Source : ....

Total of previous month : [   ]

Arrivals :   + ...   – Departures : ....
Births   :   + ...   – Deaths   : ....

————————   ————————   Monthly report

        + Subtotal : ....   – Subtotal   : ....   [   ]

Average population = $\dfrac{\text{total of previous month + monthly total}}{2}$ = [   ]

AGE DISTRIBUTION

Source : ....

Methodology of data collection : Survey [ ]   Census [ ]

Date of data collection : ....

	Male	Female	0 – 4 years	5 – 14 years	15 – 44 years	≥ 45 years	Total
%							100 %
Number							

Medical staff

The "title" (diploma, qualification) of each member of the medical staff should be indexed in the table below :

	Total	Expatriates	Nationals	Refugees
Doctors (M.D.				
Nurses				
Midwives				
Medical auxiliaries (curative)				
Lab. technician				
Community health workers (preventive)				
Village birth attendants				
Other : dentists, surgeons, ophthalmologists, pharmacists				
Traditionnal healer				
Temporary staff...				
Others (specify) : – – – – –				

Mortality

The data collection should be carried out by the administration in charge of the civilian status in order to obtain the most representative date (counting death that occured outside of health structures).

The personnel in charge of death records (political authorities, administrative, religious...) should be trained. This training consists of describing the most frequent pathologies and how to create a new file. One is only concerned with the primary cause of death.

Source of data collection : ....

Table : ....

Possible cause of death	Age						Total
	Under 1 month	1 – 11 months	0 – 4 years	5 – 14 years	15 – 44 years	≥ 45 years	
Respiratory disease							
Diarrhea							
Malaria							
Measles							
Pregnancy related deaths							
Neonatal deaths							
Trauma							
Others (specify) : – – – –							
Non documented deaths (unknown cause)							
TOTAL							

Morbidity

Record of new cases diagnosed (for the index definitions, see the following 2 pages).

New cases	0 – 4 years	5 – 14 years	15 – 44 years	≥ 45 years	Total
Upper respiratory tract infections					
Lower respiratory tract infections					
Malaria					
Measles					
Eye infections					
Watery diarrhea					
Bloody diarrhea					
Skin infections					
Sexually transmitted diseases					
Jaundice					
Urinary tract infections					
T.B. : new cases					
Meningitis					
Traumas and burns					
Others (specify) : – – – –					
Refered to hospital					
Reconsultations for one of above causes					
Total					

Rules for morbidity data collection

– The information is collected at the O.P.D. by physicians, nurses, medical auxiliaries ; the medical staff will be supervised to make sure that definitions are respected.

– **Only the new cases are recorded** : patients consulting again for the same reason, in the same month, will be recorded at the index "reconsultation".

– The diagnosis is the one mentioned at the consultation (**only one diagnosis per patient**).

Definition of the table index

– *Fever* is defined as temperature > 38°C (axilla).

– *Upper respiratory tract infections* : any nose ear throat infection (N.E.T.) (sinusitis, cold, otitis, pharyngitis, laryngitis…).

– *Lower respiratory tract infections* : any infectious episode below the larynx (bronchitis, pneumonia, bronchiolitis…).

– *Malaria* : any fever (complicated or not), related to malaria (specify the definition : clinical or proven by microscopic examiniation).

– *Measles* : fever, ± rhinopharyngitis, ± conjunctivitis, + one of the two following signs :
  • koplick's spots
  • skin eruption

– *Eye infection* : unilateral or bilateral conjunctival inflammation or infection of any other part of the eye : conjunctivitis, trachoma, keratitis…

– *Diarrhea* : any episode with more than 3 watery stools per day.
  • watery : is an estimation frequency of viral and choleriform diarrhea.
  • bloody : estimates the frequency of entero-invasive diarrhea (bacillary and amœbic dysenteria).

– *Cutaneous infection* : any cutaneous infection due to a bacterial (impetigo, pyodermitis, abscess), viral (zona, herpes…), mycosal (ring worm…) or parasitic (scabies) infection.

– *Sexually transmitted disease* : genital infections, ulcerative or discharging (vaginitis, urethritis), apparently related to sexual contamination.

– *Obstructive jaundice* : yellow conjunctivitis, discolored stools, discolored urine and associated signs. It estimates the frequency of hepatitis.

– **Urinary tract infections** : burning on micturition <u>associated</u> with pollakiuria, whether there is fever, lumbar pain or not.

– **Tuberculosis** : the new cases begin their treatment during the month of diagnosis (bacteriological positive Ziehl's colouration for the pulmonary TB).

– **Meningitis** : any meningeal syndrome with fever, diagnosed by a physician.

– **Trauma and burns** : any consultation related to trauma (fight, fall, burn, wound...).

– **Others** : tetanus, poliomyelitis, diphtheria, whooping cough, typhus, leprosy, trypanosomiasis... adapt according to the situation.
Each of these supplementary itemps will have to be defined by the team and the definition will be added to the one above.

List of essential drugs of WHO
(7th list, 1992)

1. Anaesthetics

1.1 GENERAL ANAESTHETICS AND OXYGEN

Diazepam (1b, 2)
Ether, anaesthetic (2)
Halothane (2)
Ketamine (2)
Nitrous oxide (2)
Oxygen
Δ Thiopental (2)

1.2 LOCAL ANAESTHETICS

Δ Bupivacaine (2,9)
Δ Lidocaine

1.3 PREOPERATIVE MEDICATION

Atropine
Chloral hydrate
Δ Diazepam (1b)
Δ Morphine (1a)
Δ Promethazine

2. Analgesics, anti-pyretics, non-steroidal anti-inflammatory drugs and drugs used to treat gout

2.1 NON-OPIOIDS

Acetylsalicylic acid
Allopurinol (4)
Colchicine (7)
Δ Ibuprofen
Δ Indometacin
Paracetamol

2.2 OPIOID ANALGESICS

Δ Codeine (1a)
Δ Morphine (1a)
Δ Pethidine (A) (1a, 4)

3. Antiallergics and drugs used in anaphylaxis

Δ Chlorphenamine
Δ Dexamethasone
Epinephrine
Hydrocortisone
Δ Prednisolone

4. Antidotes and other substances used in poisonings

4.1 GENERAL

Δ Charcoal, activated
Ipecacuanha

4.2 SPECIFIC

Atropine
Deferoxamine
Dimercaprol (2)
Δ Methionine
Methylthioninium chloride (methylene blue)
Naloxone
Penicillamine (2)
Potassium ferric hexacyanoferrate (II) 2H₂O (Prussian blue)
Sodium calcium edetate (2)
Sodium nitrite
Sodium thiosulfate

5. Antiepileptics

Carbamazepine
Δ Diazepam (1b)
Ethosuximide
Phenobarbital (1b)
Phenytoin
Valproic acid (7)

6. Anti-infective drugs

6.1 ANTHELMINTHICS

6.1.1 Intestinal anthelminthics

Levamisole (8)
Δ Mebendazole
Niclosamide
Piperazine
Praziquantel
Pyrantel
Tiabendazole

6.1.2 Specific anthelminthics

Albendazole

6.1.3 Antifilarials

Diethylcarbamazine
Ivermectin
Suramin sodium (2, 7)

6.1.4 Antischistosomals

Metrifonate
Oxamniquine
Praziquantel

6.2 ANTIBACTERIALS

6.2.1 Penicillins

Δ Amoxicillin (4)
Ampicillie (4)
Benzathine Benzyl penicillin (5)
Benzylpenicillin
Δ Cloxacillin
Phenoxymethyl penicillin
Δ Piperacillin
Procaine Benzylpenicillin

6.2.2 Other antibacterials

Δ Chloramphenicol (7)
Ciprofloxacin (B)
Clindamycin (B)
Doxycycline (B) (5, 6)
Δ Erythromycin
Δ Gentamicin (2, 4, 7)
Δ Metronidazole
Nitrofurantoin (B) (4, 7)
Spectinomycin (8)
Δ Sulfadimidine (4)
Δ Sulfamethoxazole + trimethoprim (4)
Δ Tetracycline
Trimethoprim (B)

6.2.3 Antileprosy drugs

Clofazimine
Dapsone
Rifampicin

6.2.4 Antituberculosis drugs

Ethambutol (4)
Isoniazid
Pyrazinamide
Rifampicin
Rifampicin + isoniazid
Streptomycin (4)
Thioacetazone + isoniazid (A) (7)

6.3 ANTIFUNGAL DRUGS

Amphotericin B (4)
Flucytosine (B) (4, 8)
Griseofulvin

6.3 ANTIFUNGAL DRUGS
(continued)
Ketoconazole (2)
Nystatin

6.4 ANTIPROTOZOAL DRUGS

6.4.1 Antiamoebic and
antigiardiasis drugs
Chloroquine (B)
Δ Diloxanide
Δ Metronidazole

6.4.2 Antileishmaniasis drugs
Δ Meglumine antimoniate
Pentamidine (5)

6.4.3 Antimalarial drugs

a) For curative treatment
Δ Chloroquine
Mefloquine (B)
Primaquine
Quinine
Δ Tétracycline (B)
Δ Sulfadoxine
+ pyrimethamine (B)

b) For prophylaxis
Chloroquine
Mefloquine (B)
Proguanil

6.4.4 Antitrypanosomal drugs

a) African trypanosomiasis
Eflornithine (C)
Melarsoprol (5)
Pentamidine (5)
Suramin sodium

b) American trypanosomiasis
Benzonidazole (7)
Nifurtimox (2, 8)

6.5 INSECT REPELLENTS
Diethyltoluamide

7. Antimigraine drugs

7.1 FOR TREATMENT OF ACUTE ATTACK
Acetylsalicylic acid
Ergotamine (7)
Paracetamol

7.2 FOR PROPHYLAXIS
Δ Propanolol

8. Antineoplastic and immunosuppressant drugs

8.1 IMMUNOSUPPRESSANT DRUGS
Δ Azathioprine (2)
Ciclosporin (2)

8.2 CYTOTOXIC DRUGS
Bleomycin (2)
Calcium folinate (C) (2)
Cisplatin (2)
Cyclophosphamide (2)
Cytarabine (2)
Dacarbazine (2)
Dactinomycin (2)
Δ Doxorubicin (2)
Etoposide (2)
Fluorouracil (2)
Mercaptopurine (2)
Methotrexate (2)
Procarbazine
Vinblastine (2)
Vincristine (2)

8.3 HORMONES AND ANTIHORMONES
Δ Dexamethasone
Δ Ethinylestradiol
Δ Prednisolone
Tamoxifen

9. Antiparkinsonism drugs
Δ Biperiden
Levodopa
+ Δ Carbidopa (5, 6)

10. Drugs affecting the blood

10.1 ANTIANAEMIA DRUGS
Ferrous salt
Ferrous salt + Folic acid
Folic acid (2)
Hydroxocobalamin (2)
Δ Iron dextran (B) (5)

10.2 DRUGS AFFECTING COAGULATION
Desmopressin (8)
Heparin
Phytomenadione
Protamine sulfate
Δ Warfarin (2, 6)

11. Blood products and plasma substitutes

11.1 PLASMA SUBSTITUTES
Δ Dextran 70
Δ Polygeline

11.2 PLASMA FRACTIONS FOR SPECIFIC USES
Albumin, human (2, 8)
Factor VIII concentrate (C) (2, 8)
Factor IX complex concentrate (C) (2, 8)

12. Cardiovascular drugs

12.1 ANTIANGINAL DRUGS
Atenolol (B)
Glyceryl trinitrate
Δ Isosorbide dinitrate
Δ Nifedipine
Δ Propranolol

12.2 ANTIDYSRHYTHMIC DRUGS
Atenolol (B)
Lidocaine
Δ Procainamide (B)
Δ Propranolol
Δ Quinidine (A)
Verapamil (8)

12.3 ANTIHYPERTENSIVE DRUGS
Atenolol (B)
Δ Captopril (B)
Δ Hydralazine
Δ Hydrochlorothiazide
Methyldopa (B) (7)
Δ Nifedipine
Δ Sodium nitroprusside (C) (2, 8)
Δ Propranolol
Δ Reserpine (A)

12.4 CARDIAC GLYCOSIDES
Digitoxin (B) (6)
Digoxin (4)

12.5 DRUGS USED IN VASCULAR SHOCK
Dopamine

12.6 ANTITHROMBOTIC DRUGS
Acetylsalicylic acid
Streptokinase (C)

13. Dermatological drugs

13.1 ANTIFUNGAL DRUGS (TOPICAL)

Benzoic acid
  + salicylic acid
Δ Miconazole
Nystatin
Sodium thiosulfate
Selenium sulfide (C)

13.2 ANTI-INFECTIVE DRUGS

Δ Methylrosanilinium chloride
     (gentian violet)
Mupirocin
Δ Neomycin + Δ Bacitracin
Silver sulfadiazine

13.3 ANTI-INFLAMMATORY AND ANTIPRURITIC DRUGS

Δ Betamethasone (3)
Δ Calamine lotion
Δ Hydrocortisone

13.4 ASTRINGENT DRUGS

Aluminium diacetate

13.5 KERATOPLASTIC AND KERATOLYTIC DRUGS

Salicylic acid
Dithranol
Fluorouracil
Coal tar
Benzoyl peroxide
Δ Podophyllum resin (7)

13.6 SCABICIDES AND PEDICULICIDES

Benzyl benzoate
Permethrin

13.7 ULTRAVIOLET-BLOCKING AGENTS

Δ Benzophenones, sun
     protection factor 15 (C)
p-aminobenzoic acid, sun
     protection factor 15 (C)
Δ Zinc oxide (C)

14. Diagnostic agents

14.1 OPHTHALMIC DRUGS

Fluorescein
Δ Tropicamide

14.2 RADIOCONTRAST MEDIA

Δ Amidotrizoate
Barium sulfate
Δ Iopanoic acid
Δ Meglumine iotroxate (C)
Δ Propyliodone

15. Disinfectants and antiseptics

15.1 ANTISEPTICS

Δ Chlorhexidine
Hydrogen peroxide
Δ Iodine

15.2 DISINFECTANTS

Calcium hypochlorite
Glutaral

16. Diuretics

Δ Amiloride (4, 7, 8)
Δ Furosemide
Δ Hydrochlorothiazide
Mannitol (C)
Spironolactone (C)

17. Gastrointestinal drugs

17.1 ANTACIDS AND OTHER ANTIULCER DRUGS

Δ Cimetidine
Aluminium hydroxide
Magnesium hydroxide

17.2 ANTIEMETIC DRUGS

Metoclopramide
Δ Promethazine

17.3 ANTIHAEMORRHOIDAL DRUGS

Δ Local anaesthetic, astringent
     and antiinflammatory
     drug

17.4 ANTI-INFLAMMATORY DRUGS

Hydrocortisone
Sulfasalazine (2)

17.5 ANTISPASMODIC DRUGS

Δ Atropine

17.6 CATHARTIC DRUGS

Δ Senna

17.7 DRUGS USED IN DIARRHEA

17.7.1 Oral rehydration

Oral rehydration salts
(for glucose-electrolyte
solution) :
  Sodium chloride 3.5 g/l
  Potassium chloride 1.5 g/l
  Trisodium citrate dihydrate
    2.9 g/l
  Glucose 20 g/l

17.7.2 Antidiarrheal (symptomatic) drugs

Δ Codeine (1a)

18. Hormones, other endocrine drugs and contraceptives

18.1 ADRENAL HORMONES AND SYNTHETIC SUBSTITUTES

Δ Dexamethasone
Fludrocortisone (C)
Hydrocortisone
Δ Prednisolone

18.2 ANDROGENS

Testosterone (C)

18.3 CONTRACEPTIVES

Depot medroxyprogesterone
  acetate (B) (7, 8)
Δ Ethinylestradiol
  + Δ levonorgestrel
Δ Ethinylestradiol
  + Δ Norethisterone
Δ Norethisterone (B)
Norethisterone enantate
  (B) (7, 8)

18.4 ESTROGENS

Δ Ethinylestradiol

18.5 INSULINS AND OTHER ANTIDIABETIC AGENTS

Insulin injection (soluble)
Intermediate-acting insulin
Δ Tolbutamide

18.6 OVULATION INDUCERS

Δ Clomifene (C) (2, 8)

18.7 PROGESTOGENS

Norethisterone

18.8 THYROID HORMONES AND ANTITHYROID DRUGS
Levothyroxine
Potassium iodide
Δ Propylthiouracile

19. Immunologicals

19.1 DIAGNOSTIC AGENTS
Tuberculin, purified protein derivative (PPD)

19.2 SERA AND IMMUNOGLOBULINS
Anti-D immunoglobulin (human)
Antiscorpion sera
Δ Antitetanus immunoglobulin (human)
Antivenom sera
Diphtheria antitoxin
Immunoglobulin, human normal (2)
Δ Rabies immunoglobulin

19.3 VACCINES

19.3.1 <u>For universal immunization</u>
BCG vaccine (dried)
Diphtheria-pertussis-tetanus vaccine
Diphtheria-tetanus vaccine
Measles-mumps-rubella vaccine
Measles vaccine
Poliomyelitis vaccine (inactivated)
Poliomyelitis vaccine (live attenuated)
Tetanus vaccine

19.3.2 <u>For specific groups of individuals</u>
Hepatitis B vaccine
Influenza vaccine
Meningococcal vaccine
Rabies vaccine
Rubella vaccine
Typhoid vaccine
Yellow fever vaccine

20. Muscle relaxants (peripherally acting) and cholinesterase inhibitors

Δ Gallamine (2)
Δ Neostigmine

Pyridostigmine (B) (2, 8)
Suxamethonium (2)
Vecuronium bromide (C)

21. Ophthalmological preparations

21.1 ANTI-INFECTIVE AGENTS
Δ Gentamicin
Δ Idoxuridine
Silver nitrate
Δ Tetracycline

21.2 ANTI-INFLAMMATORY AGENTS
Δ Prednisolone

21.3 LOCAL ANAESTHETICS
Δ Tetracaine

21.4 MYOTICS AND ANTIGLAUCOMA DRUGS
Aeétazolamide
Δ Pilocarpine
Δ Timolol

21.5 MYDRIATICS
Atropine
Epinephrine (A)

22. Oxytocics and antioxytocics

22.1 OXYTOCICS
Δ Ergometrine
Oxytocin

22.2 ANTIOXYTOCICS
Δ Salbutamol (2)

23. Peritoneal dialysis solution

Intraperitoneal dialysis solution (of appropriate composition)

24. Psychotherapeutic drugs

Δ Amitriptyline
Δ Chlorpromazine
Δ Diazepam (1b)
Δ Fluphenazine (5)
Δ Haloperidol
Lithium carbonate (2, 4)

25. Drugs acting on the respiratory tract

25.1 ANTIASTHMATIC DRUGS
Δ Cromoglicic acid (B)
Δ Aminophylline (2)
Beclometasone
Ephedrine (A)
Epinephrine
Δ Salbutamol

25.2 ANTITUSSIVES
Δ Codeine (1a)

26. Solutions correcting water, electrolyte and acid-base disturbances

26.1 ORAL REHYDRATION
Oral rehydration salts (for glucose-electrolyte solution)
Potassium chloride

26.2 PARENTERAL
Δ Compound solution of sodium lactate
Glucose
Glucose with sodium chloride
Potassium chloride (2)
Sodium chloride
Sodium hydrogen carbonate

26.3 MISCELLANEOUS
Water for injection

27. Vitamins and minerals

Ascorbic acid (C)
Calcium gluconate (C) (2, 8)
Δ Ergocalciferol
Iodine
Δ Nicotinamide
Pyridoxine
Δ Retinol
Riboflavin
Sodium fluoride (8)
Thiamine

Many drugs included in the list are preceded by a square symbol (Δ) to indicate that they represent an example of a therapeutic group and that various drugs could serve as alternatives.

Numbers in parentheses following the drug names indicate :

(1) Drugs subject to international control under : a) the Single Convention on Narcotic Drugs (1961), b) the Convention on Psychotropic Substances (1971), or c) the Convention on Illicit Traffic in Narcotic Drugs and Psychotropic Substances (1988).

(2) Specific expertise, diagnostic precision or special equipment required for proper use.

(3) Greater potency or efficacy.

(4) In renal insufficiency, contraindicated or dosage adjustments necessary.

(5) To improve compliance.

(6) Special pharmacokinetic properties.

(7) Adverse effects diminish benefit/risk ratio.

(8) Limited indications or narrow spectrum of activity.

(9) For epidural anaesthesia.

Letters in parentheses after the drug names indicate the reasons for the inclusion of complementary drugs :

(A) When drugs in the main list cannot be made available.

(B) When drugs in the main list are known to be ineffective or inappropriate for a given individual.

(C) For use in rare disorders or in exceptional circumstances.

The New Emergency Health Kit
(WHO)

Lists of drugs and medical supplies for a population of 10,000 persons for approximately 3 months

List of contents

Introduction

Chapter 1 : Essential drugs and supplies in emergency situations

Chapter 2 : Comments on the selection of drugs, medical supplies and equipment included in the kit

Chapter 3 : Composition of the New Emergency Health Kit

Annexes : 1. Basic unit : treatment guidelines

2. Evaluation and treatment of diarrhoea
2a Assessment of diarrhoea patients for dehydration
2b Treatment plan A to treat diarrhoea at home
2c Treatment plan B to treat dehydration
2d Treatment plan C to treat severe dehydration quickly

3. Management of the child with cough or difficult breathing
3a The child aged less than two months
3b The child aged two months to five years
3c Treatment instructions

4. Sample monthly activity report

5. Sample health card

6. Guidelines for suppliers

7. Useful addresses

Introduction

In recent years the various organizations and agencies of the United Nations system have been called upon to respond to an increasing number of large-scale emergencies and disasters, many of which pose a serious threat to health. Much of the assistance provided in such situations by donor agencies, governments, voluntary organizations and others is in the form of drugs and medical supplies. But the practical impact of this aid is often diminished because requests do not reflect the real needs or because these have not been adequately assessed. This can result in donations of unsorted, unsuitable and unintelligibly labelled drugs, or the provision of products which have passed their expiry date. Such problems are often compounded by delays in delivery and customs clearance.

The World Health Organization, which is the directing and coordinating authority for international health work within the United Nations system, took up the question of how emergency response could be facilitated. After several years of study, field testing and modifications, standard lists of essential drugs and medical supplies for use in an emergency were developed. The aim was to encourage the standardization of drugs and medical supplies used in an emergency to permit a swift and effective response with supplies that meet priority health needs. A further goal was to promote disaster preparedness since such standardization means that kits of essential items can be kept in readiness to meet urgent requirements.

The WHO Emergency Health Kit, which resulted from this work, was originally developed in collaboration with the Office of the United Nations High Commissioner for Refugees (UNHCR) and the London School of Hygiene and Tropical Medicine. It has now been revised in collaboration between the Action Programme on Essential Drugs (WHO, Geneva), the Emergency Preparedness and Response Unit (WHO, Geneva), the unit of Pharmaceuticals (WHO, Geneva), the Office of the United Nations High Commissioner for Refugees, UNICEF, Médecins Sans Frontières, the League of Red Cross and Red Crescent Societies (Geneva), the Christian Medical Commission of the World Council of Churches and the International Committee of the Red Cross. A review of the experience of previous users of the kit, prepared by the London School of Hygiene and Tropical Medicine, as well as field experience of UNICEF and Médecins Sans Frontières, were also considered during the revision. Major suppliers of the kit were consulted on the specifications of its contents.

The kit has now been adopted by many organizations and national authorities as a reliable, standardized, inexpensive, appropriate and quickly available source of the essential drugs and health equipment urgently needed in a disaster situation. Its contents are calculated to meet the needs of a population of 10,000 persons for three months. It has been renamed the : "New Emergency Health Kit" because of the number and diversity of United Nations agencies and other bodies which have adopted this list of drugs and medical supplies for their emergency operations and which participated in its revision.

This booklet provides background information on the development of the kit, a description of its contents, comments on the selection of items, treatment guidelines for prescribers and some useful checklists for suppliers and prescribers. Chapter 1 (Essential drugs and supplies in emergency situations) is intended as a general introduction for health administrators and field officers. Chapter 2 (Comments on the selection of drugs, medical supplies and equipment included in the kit) contains more technical details and is intended for prescribers.

Publication of this document was made possible by financial contributions received from the United Nations High Commissioner for Refugees, the Government of the Netherlands, the WHO Emergency Preparedness and Response Unit and the WHO Action Programme on Essential Drugs.

Chapter 1 : Essential drugs and supplies in Emergency situations

What is an Emergency ?

The term "emergency" is applied to various situations resulting from natural, political and economic disasters. The New Emergency Health Kit is not intended for the acute phase of epidemics, war, earthquake, floods, etc. but is designed to meet the needs of a population with disrupted medical facilities in the second phase of a natural or other disaster, or a displaced population without medical facilities. It has also been used in countries with acute shortages of drugs due to economic reasons.

It must be emphasized that, although supplying drugs and medical supplies in the standard kits is convenient in the second phase of an emergency, specific local requirements need to be assessed as soon as possible and further supplies must be ordered accordingly.

Quantification of drug requirements

Morbidity patterns (the relative frequency of different illnesses) may vary considerably between emergencies. For example, in emergencies where malnutrition is common morbidity rates may be very high. For this reason an estimation of drug requirements from a distance can only be approximate, although certain predictions can be made based on past experience. For the present kit estimates have been based on the average morbidity patterns and the use of standard treatment guidelines. The quantities of drugs supplied will therefore only be adequate if prescribers follow these guidelines (given in Annexes 1-3).

Contents of the kit

The New Emergency Health Kit consists of two different sets of drugs and medical supplies, named a BASIC UNIT and a SUPPLEMENTARY UNIT[1]. To facilitate distribution to smaller health facilities on site, the quantities of drugs and medical supplies in the basic unit have been divided into ten identical units for 1,000 persons each.

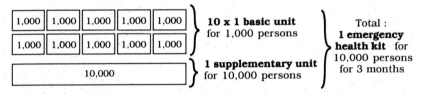

1,000	1,000	1,000	1,000	1,000
1,000	1,000	1,000	1,000	1,000

} **10 x 1 basic unit** for 1,000 persons

10,000

} **1 supplementary unit** for 10,000 persons

} Total :
1 emergency health kit for 10,000 persons for 3 months

---

[1] The previous version consisted of three lists :
A = basic drugs ; B = supplementary drugs ;
C = medical supplies and equipment for basic and supplementary lists

The BASIC UNIT contains drugs, medical supplies and some essential equipment for primary health care workers with limited training. It contains twelve drugs, none of which are injectable. Simple treatment guidelines, based on symptoms, have been developed to help the training of personnel in the proper use of the drugs. Copies of these treatment guidelines, an example of which is printed in Annexes 1-3, should be be included in each unit. Additional copies can be obtained from the Action Programme on Essential Drugs, WHO, Geneva, and from UNICEF Copenhagen (see Annex 7 for addresses).

The SUPPLEMENTARY UNIT contains drugs and medical supplies for a population of 10,000 and is to be used only by professional health workers or physicians. It does not contain any drugs or supplies from the basic units and can therefore only be used when these are available as well.

The selection and quantification of drugs for the basic and supplementary units have been based on recommendations for standard treatment regimens from technical units within WHO. A manual describing the standard treatment regimens for target diseases, developed in collaboration between Médecins sans Frontières and WHO, is available from Médecins sans Frontières at cost price and is to be included in each supplementary unit.

To facilitate identification in an emergency, one green sticker (international color code for medical items) should be placed on each parcel. The word "BASIC" should be printed on stickers for basic units.

Referral system

Health services can be decentralized by the use of basic health care clinics (the most peripheral level of health care) providing simple treatment using the basic units. Such a decentralization will : 1) increase the access of the population to curative care ; and 2) avoid overcrowding of referral facilities by solving all common health problems at the most peripheral level. Basic treatment protocols have been drawn up to allow these health workers to take the right decision on treatment or referral, according to the symptoms (see Annexes 1-3).

The first referral level should be staffed by professional health workers, usually medical assistants or doctors, who will use drugs, supplies and equipment from both the basic and the supplementary units. It should be stressed here that the basic and supplementary units have not been intended to enable these health workers to treat rare diseases or major surgical cases. For such patients a second level of referral is needed, usually a district or general hospital. Such facilities are normally part of the national health system and referral procedures are arranged with the local health authorities.

Procurement of the kit

The New Emergency Health Kit can be provided from a number of major pharmaceutical suppliers, some of which will have a permanent stock of kits ready for shipment within 48 hours. It may however be desirable to secure procurement at the regional level to reduce the cost of shipping. The procuring agency should ensure that manufacturers comply with the guidelines for quality, packaging and labelling of drugs (see Annex 6).

It is important to note that many drugs in the kit can be considered as examples of a therapeutic group, and that other drugs can often serve as alternatives. This should be taken into consideration when drugs are selected at the national level, since the choice of drugs may then be influenced by whether equivalent products are immediately available from local sources, and their comparative cost and quality. National authorities may wish to stockpile the same or equivalent drugs and supplies as part of their emergency preparedness programme. The kit can also serve as a useful baseline supply list of essential drugs for primary health care.

Donor guidelines

Whatever the source of drugs, it is very important that :
- No drugs should be sent from a donor country without a specific request, or without prior clearance by the receiving country ;
- No drugs should be sent that are not on the List of Essential Drugs of the receiving country, or, if such a national list is not available, on the WHO Model List of Essential Drugs ;
- No drugs should arrive with a future life (before expiry date) of less than one year ;
- Labelling of the drugs should be in the appropriate language(s) and should at least contain the generic name, strength, name of manufacturer and expiry date (see Annex 6) ;
- Labelling on the outside package should contain the same information, plus the total quantity of drugs in the package.

Immunization in emergency

Experience in past emergencies involving displacements of populations has shown measles to be one of the major causes of death among younger children. The disease spreads rapidly in overcrowded conditions, and serious respiratory tract infections are frequent, particularly in malnourished children. An adequate supply of essential drugs may reduce the mortality rate, but measles can be prevented by immunization. A measles immunization programme should therefore be given high priority in the early phase of an emergency. The WHO Expanded Programme on Immunization (EPI), UNICEF, the Office of the High Commissioner for Refugees (UNHCR) and OXFAM have collaborated in the development of the Emergency Immunization Kit, which may be used to set up an emergency immunization programme against measles. This kit contains cold chain and injection equipment for 5,000 immunizations and may be ordered from OXFAM. Vaccines are not included.

Post emergency needs

After the acute phase of an emergency is over and basic health needs have been covered by the basic and supplementary units, specific needs for further supplies should be assessed as soon as possible. In most cases this will necessitate a quick description and, if possible, quantification of the morbidity profile. It should characterise the most common diseases and should identify the exposed and high risk groups in the population (e.g. children below 5 years of age and pregnant women). These high risk groups should be the first target of the continuing health care programme. Any other factors that may influence requirements should also be taken into account, eg. the demographic pattern of the community, the physical condition of the individuals, seasonal variations of morbidity and mortality, the impact of improved public health measures, the local availability of drugs and other supplies, drug resistance, usual medical practice in the country, capabilities of the health workers and the effectiveness of the referral system.

Much time and money may be saved by adapting re-order forms to the specific needs of the situation and by standardizing re-order procedures for all locations and health teams, regardless of whether supplies are available locally or must be ordered from abroad.

Chapter 2 : Comments on the selection of drugs, medical supplies and equipment included in the kit

The composition of the New Emergency Health Kit is based on epidemiological data, population profiles, disease patterns and certain assumptions borne out by emergency experience. These assumptions are :

• The most peripheral level of the health care system will be staffed by health workers with only limited medical training, who will treat symptoms rather than diagnosed diseases and who will refer to the next level those patients who need more specialized treatment.

• Half of the population is 0-14 years of age.

• The average number of patients presenting themselves with the more common symptoms or diseases can be predicted.

• Standardized schedules will be used to treat these symptoms or diseases.

• The rate of referral from the basic to the next level is 10 %.

• The first referral level of health care is staffed by experienced medical assistants or medical doctors, with no or very limited facilities for inpatient care.

• If both the basic and first referral health care facilities are within reasonable reach of the target population, every individual will, on average, visit such facilities four times per year for advice or treatment. As a consequence the supplies in the kit, which are sufficient for approximately 10,000 outpatient consultations, will serve a population of 10,000 people for a period of approximately three months.

Selection of the drugs

Injectable drugs

There are no injectable drugs in the basic unit. Basic health workers with little training have usually not been taught to prescribe injections, neither are they trained to administer them. Moreover, the most common diseases in their uncomplicated form do not generally require an injectable drug. Any patient who needs an injection must be referred to the first referral level.

Antibiotics

Infectious bacterial diseases are common at all levels of health care, including the most peripheral, and basic health workers should therefore have the possiblity to prescribe an antibiotic. However, many basic health workers have not been trained to prescribe antibiotics in a rational way. Cotrimoxazole is the only antibiotic included in the basic unit, and this will enable the health worker to concentrate on taking the right decision between prescribing an antibiotic or not, rather than on the choice between several antibiotics. Cotrimoxazole has been selected because it is active against the most common bacteria found in the field, especially S. pneumoniæ and H. influenzæ for acute respiratory infections. It is also stable under tropical conditions, needs to be taken only twice daily and its side-effects (exfoliative dermatitis or bone marrow depression) are uncommon. In addition to this it is less expensive than other antibiotics. The risk of increasing bacterial resistance must be reduced by rational prescribing practice.

Drugs not included in the kit

The kit includes neither the common vaccines nor any drugs against communicable diseases such as tuberculosis or leprosy. The vaccines needed and any plans for an expanded programme on immunization should be discussed with the national authorities as soon as possible ; the same applies for programmes to combat communicable diseases. In general no special programme should be initiated unless there is sufficient guarantee for its continuation over a longer period.

In addition, drugs in the kit do not cover some specific health problems occurring in certain geographical areas, e.g. specific resistant malaria strains.

Selection of renewable supplies

Syringes and needles

Considering the risk of direct contamination with hepatitis and AIDS during handling, needles are dangerous items. The health risk for the staff should be limited by the following means :
• Limiting the number of injections ;
• Using disposable needles only ;
• Strictly following the destruction procedures for disposable material.

It is less dangerous to handle syringes than needles. For this reason a system with resterilisable nylon syringes and disposable needles has been chosen for the supplementary unit. However, in the very first stage, when sterilization procedures are not yet established, some provision will be necessary for giving injections by means of fully disposable materials. A small number of disposable syringes are therefore provided in the supplementary unit and their destruction should be supervised by the person in charge.

The New Emergency Health Kit – WHO

Gloves

Disposable protective gloves are provided in the basic unit to protect health workers against possible infection during dressings or handling of infected materials. In any case a dressing should be applied or changed with the instruments provided in the kit. Surgical gloves, which should be resterilizable, are supplied in the supplementary unit. They are to be used for deliveries, sutures and minor surgery, all under medical supervision.

Selection of equipment

Resuscitation / Surgical instruments

The kit has been designed for general medicine under primitive conditions, and for that reason no equipment for resuscitation or major surgery has been included. In situations of war, earthquakes or epidemics, specialised teams with medical equipment and supplies will be required.

Sterilization

A complete sterilization set is provided in the kit. The basic units contain two small drums each for sterile dressing materials. Two drums are included to enable the alternate sterilization of one at the first referral level while the other is being used in the peripheral facility. The supplementary unit contains a kerosene stove and two pressure sterilizers, a small one for sterilizing 2 ml and 5 ml syringes, and a larger one for the small drums with dressing materials and the instrument sets.

Dilution and storage of liquids

The kit contains several plastic bottles and a few large disposable syringes which are needed to dilute and store liquids (e.g. benzyl benzoate, chlorhexidine and gentian violet solution).

Water supply

The kit contains several items to help provide for clean water at the health facility. Each basic unit contains a 20 litre foldable jerrycan and a plastic bucket. The supplementary unit contains a water filter with candles and 2.5 kg of chloramine powder to chlorinate the water.

Chapter 3 : Composition of the New Emergency Health Kit

The New Emergency Health Kit consists of ten basic units and one supplementary unit.

10 basic units (for basic health workers) for a population of 10,000 persons for 3 months (1 basic unit for 1,000 persons for 3 months). The unit contains drugs, renewable supplies and basic equipment packed in one carton.

1 supplementary unit (for physicians and senior health workers), for a population of 10,000 people for 3 months. One supplementary unit contains :
– drugs (approximately 130 kg)
– essential infusions (approximately 180 kg)
– renewable supplies (approximately 60 kg)
– equipment (approximately 40 kg)

NB : The supplementary unit does not contain any drugs and medical supplies from the basic unit. To be operational, the supplementary unit should be used together with ten basic units.

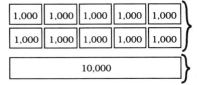

1,000	1,000	1,000	1,000	1,000
1,000	1,000	1,000	1,000	1,000

10 x 1 basic unit
10 x (45 kg/0.20 m³)

10,000

1 supplementary unit
approx. 410 kg - 2 m³

1 emergency health kit for 10,000 persons for 3 months approx. 860 kg 4 m³

Basic unit (for 1,000 persons for 3 months)

Drugs

Acetylsalicylic acid, tab 300 mg ....tab	3,000
Aluminium hydroxyde, tab 500 mg ....tab	1,000
1) Benzyl benzoate, lotion 25 % ....bottle 1 litre	1
2) Chlorhexidine (5%)..bottle 1 litre	1
Chloroquine, tab 150 mg base ....tab	2,000
Ferrous Sulfate + Folic Acid, tab 200 + 0.25 mg..tab	2,000
Gentian Violet, powder..25 g	4
Mebendazole, tab 100 mg...tab	500
ORS (Oral Rehydration Salts) ....sachet for 1 litre	200
Paracetamol, tab 100 mg..tab	1,000
Sulfamethoxazole + Trimetoprim, tab 400 + 80mg (cotrimoxazole)...............tab	2,000
Tetracycline eye ointment 1 % ....tube 5 g	50

Renewable supplies

Absorbent cotton wool ....kg	1
Adhesive tape 2.5 cm x 5 m..roll	30
Bar of soap (100-200 g) ....bar	10
Elastic bandage (crepe) 7.5 cm x 10 m ....unit	20
Gauze bandage 7.5 cm x 10 m,..roll	100
Gauze compress 10 x 10 cm, 12 ply, nonsterile..unit	500
Ballpen, blue or black..unit	10
Exercise book A4..unit	4
3) Health card + plastic sachet ....unit	500
Small plastic bag for drugs..unit	2,000
Notepad A6 ....unit	10
Thermometer (oral/rectal) Celsius / Fahrenheit...unit	6
Protective glove, nonsterile, disposable ....unit	100
4) *Treatment guidelines for basic list*..unit	2

Equipment

Nail brush, plastic, autoclavable ....unit	2
Bucket, plastic, approx. 20 litres ....unit	1
Gallipot, stainless steel, 100 ml...unit	1

---

1) *According to WHO recommendations Benzyl benzoate solution 25 % concentration is being supplied. The use of 90 % concentration is not recommended.*

2) *Chlorhexidine 20 % needs distilled water for dilution, otherwise precipitation may occur. 5 % solution is WHO standard. Alternatives include the combination of chlorhexidine 1.5 % and cetrimide 15 %.*

3) *For a sample health card, see Annex 4.*

4) *For sample treatment guidelines, see Annexes 1, 2 and 3.*

Kidney dish, stainless steel, approx. 26 x 14 cm ....unit	1
1) Dressing set (3 instruments + box)..unit	2
Dressing tray, stainless steel, approx. 30 x 15 x 3 cm....................................unit	1
Drum for compresses approx. 15 cm H, Ø 14 cm ....unit	2
Foldable jerrycan, 20 litres...unit	1
Forceps Kocher, no teeth, 12-14 cm ....unit	2
Plastic bottle, 1 litre ....unit	3
Syringe Luer, disposable, 10 ml..unit	1
Plastic bottle, 125 ml...unit	1
Scissors straight/blunt, 12-14 cm ....unit	2

---

1) *Dressing set (3 instruments + box) :*
   - *1 stainless steel box approx. 17 x 7 x 3 cm*
   - *1 pair surgical scissors, sharp/blunt, 12-14 cm*
   - *1 Kocher forceps, no teeth, straight, 12-14 cm*
   - *1 dissecting forceps, no teeth, 12-14 cm*

Supplementary unit (for 10,000 persons for 3 months)

Drugs

Anaesthesics

Ketamine, inj. 50 mg/ml ....10 ml / vial	25
1) Lidocaïne, inj. 1 % ....20 ml / vial	50

Analgesics

2) Pentazocine, inj. 30 mg/ml...1 ml / ampoule	50
3) Probenecid, tab 500 mg...tab	500

Recall from basic unit :
Acetyl salicyclic acid, tab 300 mg..(10 x 3,000) 30,000
Paracetamol, tab 100 mg ....(10 x 1,000) 10,000

Anti-allergics

Dexamethasone, inj. 4 mg/ml..1 ml / amp.	50
Prednisolone, tab 5 mg ....tab	100
Epinephrine (adrenaline), see "respiratory tract"	

Anti-epileptics

Diazepam, inj. 5 mg/ml...2 ml / ampoule	200
Phenobarbital, tab 50 mg..tab	1,000

Anti-infective drugs

4) Ampicillin, tab 250 mg ....tab	2,000
4) Ampicillin, inj. 500 mg /vial ....vial	200
Benzathine benzylpenicillin, inj. 2.4 MIU / vial.............................vial	50
Chloramphenicol, caps 250 mg..caps	2,000
Chloramphenicol, inj. 1 g / vial ....vial	500
Metronidazole, tab 250 mg..tab	2,000
5) Nystatin, non-coated tablet..100,000 IU / tab	2,000
Phenoxymethylpenicillin, tab 250 mg..tab	4,000
6) Procaïn benzylpenicillin, inj. 3-4 MU / vial...................................vial	1,000

---

1) *20 ml vials are preferred, although 50 ml vials may be used as an alternative.*

2) *Because of narcotic drugs regulation, pentazocine has been chosen as an alternative to morphine or pethidine.*

3) *To be used with penicillin in the treatment of gonorrhoea.*

4) *Ampicillin tablets and injections to be used only in neonates and pregnant women.*

5) *For the treatment of oral candidiasis.*

6) *The combination of procaine benzylpenicillin 3 MU and benzylpenicillin 1 MU (procaine penicillin fortified) is used in many countries and may be included as an alternative.*

1) Quinine, inj. 300 mg/ml ....2 ml / amp. | 100
Quinine sulfate, tab 300 mg ....tab | 3,000
2) Sulfadoxine + pyrimethamine, tab 500 mg + 25 mg ....tab | 300
3) Tetracycline, caps or tab 250 mg...caps or tab | 2,000

Recall from basic unit :
Mebendazole, tab 100 mg ....(10 x 500) 5,000
Cotrimoxazole, tab 400 + 80 mg...(10 x 2,000) 20,000
Chloroquine, tab 150 mg...(10 x 2,000) 20,000

Blood, drugs affecting the

Folic acid, tab 1 mg .... | 5,000

Recall from basic unit :
Ferrous sulfate + Folic acid, tab 200 + 0.25 mg ....(10 x 2,000) 20,000

Cardiovascular drugs

4) Methyldopa, tab 250 mg...tab | 500
Hydralazine, inj. 20 mg/ml...1 ml / amp. | 20

Dermatological

5) Polyvidone iodine 10 %, sol., 500 ml...bottle | 4
Zinc oxyde 10 % ointment...kg | 2
Benzoic acid 6 % + salicylic acid 3 % ointment..............................kg | 1

Recall from basic unit :
Tetracycline eye ointment, 1 %...(10 x 50) 500
Gentian violet, powder 25 g...(10 x 4) 40
Benzyl benzoate, lotion 25 %, litre...(10 x 1) 10

Diuretics

Furosemide, inj. 10 mg/ml..2 ml / amp. | 20
Furosemide, tab 40 mg ....tab | 200

Gastro-intestinal drugs

Promethazine, tab 25 mg..tab | 500
Promethazine, inj. 25 mg/ml ....2 ml / amp. | 50
Atropine, inj. 1 mg/ml...1 ml / amp. | 50

Recall from basic unit :
Aluminium hydroxyde, tab 500 mg ....(10 x 1,000) 10,000

---

1) *For the treatment of cerebral and resistant malaria cases. Intravenous injection of quinine must always be diluted in 500 ml glucose 5 %.*

2) *For the treatment of resistant malaria strains (check national protocols).*

3) *For the treatment of cholera and chlamydia infections.*

4) *For the treatment of hypertension in pregnancy.*

5) *Polyvidone iodine has been chosen because the use of iodine tincture in hot climates may result in toxic concentrations of iodine by partial evaporation of the alcohol.*

Oxtocics

Ergometrine maleate, inj. 0.2 mg/ml..1 ml / amp.	200

Psychotherapeutic drugs

Chlorpromazine, inj. 25 mg/ml...2 ml / amp.	20

Respiratory tract, drugs acting on

Aminophylline, tab 100 mg ....tab	1,000
Aminophylline, inj. 25 mg/ml...10 ml / amp.	50
Epinephrine (adrenaline), inj. 1 mg/ml ....1 ml / amp.	50

Solutions correcting water, electrolyte and acid-base disturbances [1]

Compound solution of sodium lactate (Ringer's Lactate), inj. sol., with giving set and needle..500 ml / bag	200
2) Glucose, inj. sol. 5 %, with giving set and needle............................500 ml / bag	100
Glucose, inj. sol. 50 % ....50 ml / vial	20
Water for injection ....10 ml / plastic vial	2,000

Recall from basic unit :

ORS (Oral Rehydration Salts)..(10 x 200) 2,000

Vitamins

Retinol (Vitamin A), caps 200,000 IU ....caps	4,000
Ascorbic acid, tab 250 mg ....tab	4,000

Renewable supplies

Scalp vein infusion set, disposable, 25G (Ø 0.5 mm) ....unit	300
Scalp vein infusion set, disposable, 21G (Ø 0.8 mm) ....unit	100
IV placement canula, disposable, 18G (Ø 1.7 mm)..unit	15
IV placement canula, disposable, 22G (Ø 0.9 mm)..unit	15
Needle Luer IV, disposable, 19G (Ø 1.1 mm x 38 mm)...............................unit	1,000
Needle Luer IM, disposable, 21G (Ø 0.8 mm x 40 mm)..............................unit	2,000
Needle Luer SC, disposable, 25G (Ø 0.5 mm x 16 mm).............................unit	100
Spinal needle, disposable, 20G (64 mm - Ø 0.9 mm).....................................unit	30
Spinal needle, disposable, 23G (64 mm - Ø 0.7 mm).....................................unit	30
Syringe Luer resterilisable, nylon, 2 ml...unit	20
Syringe Luer resterilisable, nylon, 5 ml...unit	100

---

1) *Because of the weight, the quantity of infusions included in the kit is minimal. Look for local supply, once in the field.*

2) *Glucose 5 %, bag 500 ml, for dilution of quinine/injection.*

Syringe Luer resterilisable, nylon, 10 ml ....unit | 40
Syringe Luer, disposable, 2 ml ....unit | 400
Syringe Luer, disposable, 5 ml ....unit | 500
Syringe Luer, disposable, 10 ml ....unit | 200
Syringe conic connector (for feeding), 60 ml.......................................unit | 20
Feeding tube, CH5 (premature baby), disposable................................unit | 20
Feeding tube, CH8, disposable..unit | 50
Feeding tube, CH16, disposable..unit | 10
Urinary catheter (Foley), n°12, disposable...unit | 10
Urinary catheter (Foley), n°14, disposable...unit | 5
Urinary catheter (Foley), n°18, disposable...unit | 5
Surgical gloves sterile and resterilisable n°6.5 ....pair | 50
Surgical gloves sterile and resterilisable n°7.5 ....pair | 150
Surgical gloves sterile and resterilisable n°8.5 ....pair | 50

Recall from basic unit :
Protective glove, non sterile, disposable...(100 units x 10) 1,000

Sterilization test tape (for autoclave)...roll | 2
Chloramine, tabs or powder...kg | 2.5
Thermometer (oral/rectal) dual Celsius / Fahrenheit ....unit | 10
Spare bulb for otoscope ....unit | 2
Batteries R6 alkaline AA size (for otoscope) ....unit | 6

Recall from basic unit :
Thermometer (oral/rectal) celsius / fahrenheit ....(6 units x 10) 60
Ballpen, blue or black ....(10 units x 10) 100
Exercise book A4 ....(4 units x 10) 40
Health card + plastic sachet ....(500 units x 10) 5,000
Small plastic bag for drugs ....(2,000 units x 10) 20,000
Notepad A6 ....(10 units x 10) 100

Urine collecting bag with valve, 2000 ml..unit | 10
Finger stall 2 fingers, disposable...unit | 300
Suture, synthetic absorbable, braided, size DEC.2 (000) with
   cutting needle curved 3/8, 20 mm triangular ....unit | 24
Suture, synthetic absorbable, braided, size DEC.3 (00) with
   cutting needle curved 3/8, 30 mm triangular ....unit | 36
Surgical blade (surgical knives) n°22 for handle n°4 ....unit | 50
Razor blade ....unit | 100
Tongue depressor (wooden), disposable ....unit | 100
Gauze roll 90 m x 0.90 m ....roll | 3
Gauze compress 10 x 10 cm, 12 ply, sterile ....unit | 1,000

Recall from basic unit :
Absorbent cotton wool..(1 kg x 10) 10
Adhesive tape 2.5 cm x 5 m...(30 rolls x 10) 300
Bar of soap (100-200 g/bar) ....(10 bars x 10) 100
Elastic bandage (crepe) 7.5 cm x 10 m..........................(20 units x 10) 200
Gauze bandage 7.5 cm x 10 m.......................................(100 rolls x 10) 1,000
Gauze compress 10 x 10 cm, 12 ply, nonsterile ....(500 units x 10) 5,000

Equipment

Clinical stethoscope, dual cup ....unit	2
Obstetrical stethoscope (metal) ....unit	1
Sphygmomanometer (adult)..unit	1
Razor non disposable..unit	2
Scale for adult..unit	1
Scale hanging 25 kg x 100 g (Salter type) + 3 trousers ....unit	3
Tape measure..unit	5
Drum for compresses, h : 15 cm, Ø 14 cm...unit	2

Recall from basic unit :
Drum for compresses, approx. h : 15 cm, Ø 14 cm...(2 units x 10) 20

Otoscope + disposable set of pædiatric speculums..unit	1
Tourniquet ....unit	2
Dressing tray, stainless steel, approx. 30 x 15 x 3 cm.....................................unit	1
Kidney dish, stainless steel, approx. 26 x 14 cm ....unit	1
Scissors straight/blunt, 12-14 cm ....unit	2
Forceps Kocher no teeth, 12-14 cm..unit	2

Recall from basic unit :
Kidney dish, stainless steel, approx. 26 x 14 cm...(1 unit x 10) 10
Gallipot, stainless steel, 100 ml ....(1 unit x 10) 10
Dressing tray, stainless steel, approx. 30 x 15 x 3 cm..(1 unit x 10) 10
Scissors straight/blunt, 12-14 cm ....(2 units x 10) 20
Forceps Kocher, no teeth, 12-14 cm...(2 units x 10) 20

1) Abcess/suture set (7 instruments + box) ....unit	2
2) Dressing set (3 instruments + box)..unit	5

Recall from basic unit :
Dressing set (3 instruments + box) ....(2 units x 10) 20

---

1) *Abscess/suture set (7 instruments + box) :*
   - *1 stainless steel box approx. 20 x 10 x 5 cm*
   - *1 dissecting forceps, with teeth, 12-14 cm*
   - *1 Kocher forceps, with teeth, straight, 12-14 cm*
   - *1 Pean forceps, straight, 12-14 cm*
   - *1 pair surgical scissors, sharp/blunt, 12-14 cm*
   - *1 probe, 12-14 cm*
   - *1 Mayo-Hegar needle holder, 18 cm*
   - *1 handle scalpel n°4*

2) *Dressing set (3 instruments + box) :*
   - *1 stainless steel box approx. 17 x 7 x 3 cm*
   - *1 pair surgical scissors, sharp/blunt, 12-14 cm*
   - *1 Kocher forceps, no teeth, straight, 12-14 cm*
   - *1 dissecting forceps, no teeth, 12-14 cm*

Pressure sterilizer, 7.5 litres (type : Prestige 7506, double rack,
  ref. UNIPAC 01.571.00) ....unit   1
  Additional rack Public Health Care 2ml/5ml, ref.Prestige 7531 ....unit   2
Pressure sterilizer, 20-40 litres with basket (type UNIPAC 01.560.00).........unit   1
Kerosene stove, single burner (type UNIPAC 01.700.00) ....unit   2
Water filter with candles, 10-20 litres (type UNIPAC 56.199.02) ....unit   3
Nail brush, plastic, autoclavable ....unit   2

Recall from basic unit :

Plastic bottle, 1 litre ....*(3 units x 10) 30*
Syringe Luer, disposable, 10 ml ....*(1 unit x 10) 10*
Plastic bottle, 125 ml ....*(1 unit x 10) 10*
Nail brush, plastic autoclavable ....*(2 units x 10) 20*
Bucket, plastic, approx. 20 litres ....*(1 unit x 10) 10*
Foldable jerrycan, 20 litres ....*(1 unit x 10) 10*

Portable weight / height chart (UNICEF/SCF) (UNIPAC 01.455.70) ....unit   1
1) Clinical guidelines - diagnostic and treatment manual   1
1) Guide clinique et thérapeutique...   1
1) Guía clínica y terapéutica   1

---

1) *Available at cost price from Médecins Sans Frontières.*

Basic unit : treatment guidelines

These treatment guidelines are intended to give simple guidance for the training of primary health care workers using the basic unit. In the dosage guidelines, five age groups have been distinguished. When dosage is shown as 1 tab. x 2, one tablet should be taken in the morning and one before bedtime. When dosage is shown as 2 tab. x 3, two tablets should be taken in the morning, two should be taken in the middle of the day and two before bedtime.

The treatment guidelines contain the following diagnosis/symptom groups :
• Anemia
• Pain
• Diarrhoea : *see detailed diagnosis and treatment schedules in Annex 2 a-c.*
• Fever
• Respiratory tract infections : *see detailed diagnosis and treatment schedules in Annex 3.*
• Measles
• Eye
• Skin conditions
• Urinary tract infections
• Sexually transmitted disease
• Preventive care in pregnancy
• Worms

DIAGNOSIS / SYMPTOM \ WEIGHT / AGE	4 kg / 2 months	8 kg / 1 year	15 kg / 5 years	35 kg / 15 years	ADULT

➜ *Anemia*

	4 kg / 2 months	8 kg / 1 year	15 kg / 5 years	35 kg / 15 years	ADULT
Severe anemia (œdemas, dizziness, shortness of breath)		**Refer**			
Moderate anemia (pallor and tiredness)	**Refer**	*Ferrous sulfate + Folic acid* 1 tab. daily for at least 2 months	*Ferrous sulfate + Folic acid* 2 tab. daily for at least 2 months	*Ferrous sulfate + Folic acid* 3 tab. daily for at least 2 months	*Ferrous sulfate + Folic acid* 3 tab. daily for at least 2 months

➜ *Pain*

	4 kg / 2 months	8 kg / 1 year	15 kg / 5 years	35 kg / 15 years	ADULT
Pain headache, joint pain, tooth ache...		*Paracetamol* tab 100 mg 1/2 tab. x 3	*Paracetamol* tab 100 mg 1 tab. x 3	*ASA* [1][2] tab 300 mg 1 tab. x 3	*ASA* [1] tab 300 mg 2 tab. x 3
Stomach pain			**Refer**	*Aluminium hydroxide* 1/2 tab. x 3 for 3 days	*Aluminium hydroxide* 1 tab. x 3 for 3 days

[1] *ASA = Acetyl Salicylic Acid*
[2] *For children under 12 paracetamol is to be preferred because of the risk of Reye's Syndrome.*

DIAGNOSIS SYMPTOM \ WEIGHT AGE	4 kg 2 months	8 kg 1 year	15 kg 5 years	35 kg 15 years	ADULT

➔ *Diarrhoea*

Diarrhoea lasting more than 2 weeks or in malnourished or poor condition patient	Give *ORS* according to dehydration stage and **refer**				
Bloody diarrhoea[1] (check the presence of blood in the stools)	Give *ORS* according to dehydration stage and **refer**				
Diarrhoea with severe dehydration (Plan C, WHO) Annex 2d	*ORS*, 100 ml/kg as soon as possible, and **refer** patient for nasogastric tube and/or IV treatment.				
Diarrhoea with some dehydration (Plan B, WHO) Annex 2c	Treat with *ORS*, 50-100 ml/kg in first 4-6 hours, reassess the condition after 4-6 hours				
	250 ml within 6 h	500 ml within 6 h	1 litre within 6 h	2 litres within 6 h	3 litres or + within 6 h
Diarrhoea with no dehydration (Plan A, WHO) Annex 2b	- Continue to feed. - Return to health worker in case of frequent stools, increased thirst, sunken eyes, fever, or when the patient does not eat or drink normally, or does not get better.				

➔ *Fever*

Fever in malnourished or poor condition patient or when in doubt	**Refer**				
Fever with chills assuming it is malaria	**Refer**	*Chloroquine*[2] tab 150mg base 1/2 tab at once, then 1/4 tab. after 6 h, 24 h and 48 h	*Chloroquine*[2] tab 150mg base 1 tab at once, then 1/2 tab. after 6 h, 24 h and 48 h	*Chloroquine*[2] tab 150mg base 2 tab at once, then 1 tab. after 6 h, 24 h and 48 h	*Chloroquine*[2] tab 150mg base 4 tab at once, then 2 tab. after 6 h, 24 h and 48 h
Fever with cough	**Refer**	See "Respiratory tract infections"			
Fever (unspecified)	**Refer**	*Paracetamol* tab 100 mg 1/2 tab. x 3 for 1 to 3 days	*Paracetamol* tab 100 mg 1 tab. x 3 for 1 to 3 days	*ASA* [3] tab 300 mg 1 tab. x 3 for 1 to 3 days	*ASA* tab 300 mg 2 tab. x 3 for 1 to 3 days

[1] *Protocol will be established according to epidemiological data. Cotrimoxazole will usually be effective..*
[2] *Chloroquine 150 mg base is equivalent to 250 mg chloroquine phosphate or to 200 mg chloroquine sulfate.*
[3] *For children under 12 paracetamol is to be preferred because of the risk of Reye's Syndrome.*

DIAGNOSIS / SYMPTOM \ AGE / WEIGHT		4 kg / 2 months	8 kg / 1 year	15 kg / 5 years	35 kg / 15 years — ADULT

➜ *Respiratory tract infections*

Severe pneumonia Annex 3		Give the first dose of *cotrimoxazole* (see pneumonia) and **refer.**			
Pneumonia Annex 3	**Refer**	*Cotrimoxazole* tab 400 mg SMX + 80mg TMP 1/2 tab. x 2 for 5 days	*Cotrimoxazole* tab 400 mg SMX + 80mg TMP 1 tab. x 2 for 5 days	*Cotrimoxazole* tab 400 mg SMX + 80mg TMP 1 tab. x 2 for 5 days	*Cotrimoxazole* tab 400 mg SMX + 80mg TMP 2 tab. x 2 for 5 days
		Reassess after 2 days ; continue (breast) feeding, give fluids, clear the nose ; return if breathing becomes faster or more difficult, or not able to drink or condition deteriorates.			
No pneumonia : **cough or cold** Annex 3	**Refer**	*Paracetamol*[1] tab 100 mg 1/2 tab x 3 for 3 days	*Paracetamol*[1] tab 100 mg 1 tab x 3 for 3 days	*ASA*[1] tab 300 mg 1 tab x 3 for 3 days	*ASA*[1] tab 300 mg 2 tab x 3 for 3 days
		Supportive therapy : continue (breast) feeding, give fluids, clear the nose ; return if breathing becomes faster or more difficult, or not able to drink or condition deteriorates.			
Prolonged cough (over 30 days)		**Refer**			
Acute ear pain and/or **ear discharge** For **less** than 2 weeks	**Refer**	*Cotrimoxazole* tab 400 mg SMX + 80mg TMP 1/2 tab. x 2 for 5 days[1]	*Cotrimoxazole* tab 400 mg SMX + 80mg TMP 1 tab. x 2 for 5 days[1]	*Cotrimoxazole* tab 400 mg SMX + 80mg TMP 1 tab. x 2 for 5 days	*Cotrimoxazole* tab 400 mg SMX + 80mg TMP 2 tab. x 2 for 5 days
Ear discharge For **more** than 2 weeks, no pain, no fever		Clean the ear once daily by syringe without needle using lukewarm clean water. Repeat until the water comes out clean. Dry repeatedly with clean piece of cloth.			

[1] *If fever is present.*
[2] *For children under 12 paracetamol is to be preferred because of the risk of Reye's Syndrome.*

	WEIGHT	4 kg	8 kg	15 kg	35 kg	ADULT
DIAGNOSIS **SYMPTOM**	AGE	2 months	1 year	5 years	15 years	

➜ *Measles*

Measles	Treat respiratory tract disease according to symptoms. Treat conjunctivitis as "Red eyes". Treat diarrhoea according to symptoms. Continue (breast) feeding. Give *Retinol* (*vitamin A*).

➜ *Eye*

Red eyes (conjunctivitis)	Apply *Tetracycline eye ointment* 3 times a day for 7 days. If not improved after 3 days or in doubt : **refer**.

➜ *Skin conditions*

Wounds : extensive, deep or on face	**Refer**
Wounds : limited and superficial	Clean with clean water and soap or with <u>diluted</u> *Chlorhexidine solution** Apply *Gentian Violet solution*** once a day.
Severe burns (on face or very extensive)	Treat as for mild burns, and **refer**.
Mild, moderate burns	Immerse <u>immediately</u> in cold water, or use a cold wet cloth. Continue until pain ceases. Then, treat as wounds
Severe bacterial infection (with fever)	**Refer**
Mild bacterial infection	Clean with clean water and soap or <u>diluted</u> *Chlorhexidine solution** Apply *Gentian Violet solution*** twice a day. If not improved after 10 days : **refer**.
Fungal infection	Apply *Gentian Violet solution*** once a day for 5 days.
Infected scabies	Bacterial infection : clean with clean water and soap or <u>diluted</u> *Chlorhexidine solution** and apply *Gentian Violet solution*** twice a day. When infection is cured :
	Apply <u>diluted</u> *Benzyl benzoate**** once a day for 3 days Apply <u>non diluted</u> *Benzyl benzoate 25 %* once a day for 3 days
Non infected scabies	Apply <u>diluted</u> *Benzyl benzoate**** once a day for 3 days Apply <u>non diluted</u> *Benzyl benzoate 25 %* once a day for 3 days

*   *Chlorhexidine 5 % must always be diluted before use : 20 ml in 1 litre of water (take one litre plastic bottle supplied with kit. Put 20 ml of Chlorhexidine solution into the bottle using the 10 ml syringe supplied with the kit. Fill up the bottle with boiled or clean water). Chlorhexidine 1.5 % + Cetrimide 15 % solution should be use at the same dilution.*
** *Dissolve gentian violet : 0.5 % concentration = 1 tea spoon of gentian violet powder per litre of boiled/clean water.*
*** *Dilute by mixing one half litre Benzyl benzoate 25 % with one half litre clean water in the one litre plastic bottle supplied with the kit.*

The New Emergency Health Kit – WHO

	WEIGHT	4 kg	8 kg	15 kg	35 kg	ADULT
DIAGNOSIS SYMPTOM	AGE	2 months	1 year	5 years	15 years	

→ Urinary tract infection

Suspicion of urinary tract infection			Refer		

→ Sexually transmitted disease

Suspicion of sexually transmitted disease (syphilis, gonorrhœa)			Refer		

→ Preventive care in pregnancy

Anemia for treatment, see under Anemia		*Ferrous sulfate + Folic acid* 1 tab. daily, throughout pregnancy
Malaria for treatment, see under Fever		*Chloroquine*[1] tab 150mg base 2 tab weekly, throughout pregnancy

→ Worms

		15 kg	35 kg	ADULT
Roundworm Pinworm		*Mebendazole* tab 100 mg 2 tab. once	*Mebendazole* tab 100 mg 2 tab. once	*Mebendazole* tab 100 mg 2 tab. once
Hookworm		*Mebendazole* tab 100 mg 1 tab. x 2 for 3 days	*Mebendazole* tab 100 mg 1 tab. x 2 for 3 days	*Mebendazole* tab 100 mg 1 tab. x 2 for 3 days

[1] *Chloroquine 150 mg base is equivalent to 250 mg chloroquine phosphate or to 200 mg chloroquine sulfate.*

Evaluation and treatment of diarrhoea

Assessment of diarrhoea patients for dehydration

First assess your patient for dehydration			
	A	**B**	**C**
1. LOOK AT :			
CONDITION	Well, alert	Restless, irritable	Lethargic or unconscious ; floppy
EYES[1]	Normal	Sunken	Very sunken and dry
TEARS	Present	Absent	Absent
MOUTH and TONGUE[2]	Moist	Dry	Very dry
THIRST	Drinks normally, not thirsty	Thirsty, drinks eagerly	Drinks poorly or not able to drink
2. FEEL :			
SKIN PINCH[3]	Goes back quickly	Goes back slowly	Goes back very slowly
3. DECIDE :	The patient has NO SIGN OF DEHYDRATION	If the patient has two or more signs, including at least one sign, there is SOME DEHYDRATION	If the patient has two or more signs, including at least one sign, there is SEVERE DEHYDRATION
4. TREAT :	Use *Treatment plan A*	Weigh the patient, if possible, and use *Treatment plan B*	Weigh the patient and use *Treatment plan C* URGENTLY

[1] *In some infants and children the eyes normally appear somewhat sunken. It is helpful to ask the mother if the child's eyes are normal or more sunken than usual.*

[2] *Dryness of the mouth and tongue can also be palpated with a clean finger. The mouth may always be dry in a child who habitually breathes through the mouth. The mouth may be wet in a dehydrated patient owing to recent vomiting or drinking.*

[3] *The skin pinch is less useful in infants or children with marasmus (severe wasting) or kwashiorkor (severe undernutrition with œdema), or obese children.*

Source : *A manual for the treatment of diarrhoea* (WHO / CDD – 1990)

Treatment plan A to treat diarrhoea at home

Use this plan to teach the mother to :

- Continue to treat at home her child's current episode of diarrhoea.
- Give early treatment for future episodes of diarrhoea.

Explain the three rules for treating diarrhoea at home

1. GIVE THE CHILD MORE FLUIDS THAN USUAL TO PREVENT DEHYDRATION :

- Use a recommended home fluid, such as a cereal gruel. If this is not possible, give plain water.
- Use ORS solution for children described in the box overleaf.
- Give as much of these fluids as the child will take. Use the amounts shown below for ORS as a guide.
- Continue giving these fluids until the diarrhoea stops.

2. GIVE THE CHILD PLENTY OF FOOD TO PREVENT UNDERNUTRITION :

- Continue to breast-feed frequently.
- If the child is not breast-fed, give the usual milk. If the child is less than 6 months old and not yet taking solid food, dilute milk of formula with an equal amount of water for 2 days.
- If the child is 6 months or older, or already taking solid food :
  - Also give cereal or another starchy food mixed, if possible, with pulses, vegetables, and meat of fish. Add 1 or 2 teaspoonfuls of vegetable oil to each serving.
  - Give fresh fruit juice or mashed banana to provide potassium.
  - Give freshly prepared foods. Cook and mash or grind food well.
  - Encourage the child to eat : offer food at least 6 times a day.
  - Give the same foods after diarrhoea stops, and give an extra meal each day for two weeks.

3. TAKE THE CHILD TO THE HEALTH WORKER IF THE CHILD DOES NOT GET BETTER IN 3 DAYS OR DEVELOPS ANY OF THE FOLLOWING :

- Many watery stools
- Repeated vomiting
- Marked thirst

- Eating or drinking poorly
- Fever
- Blood in the stool

Children should be given ORS solutions at home, if :

- They have been on Treatment Plan B or C.
- They cannot return to the health worker if the diarrhoea gets worse.
- It is national policy to give ORS to all children who see a health worker for diarrhoea.

IF THE CHILD WILL BE GIVEN ORS SOLUTION AT HOME, SHOW THE MOTHER HOW MUCH ORS TO GIVE AFTER EACH LOOSE STOOL AND GIVE HER ENOUGH PACKETS FOR 2 DAYS :

Age	Amount of ORS to give after each loose stool	Amount of ORS to provide for use at home
Less than 24 moths	50-100 ml	500 ml/day
2 up to 10 years	100-200 ml	1,000 ml/day
10 years or more	As much as wanted	2,000 ml/day

- Describe and show the amount to be given after each stool using a local measure.

Show the mother how to mix ORS.
Show her how to give ORS :

- Give a teaspoonful every 1-2 minutes for a child under 2 years.
- Give frequent sips from a cup for an older child.
- If the child vomits, wait 10 minutes. Then give the solution more slowly (for example, a spoonful every 2-3 minutes).
- If diarrhoea continues after the ORS packets are used up, tell the mother to give other fluids as described in the first rule above or return for more ORS.

Treatment plan B to treat dehydration

APPROXIMATE AMOUNT OF ORS SOLUTION TO GIVE IN THE FIRST 4 HOURS :

Age*	Less than 4 months	4-11 months	12-23 months	2-4 years	5-14 years	15 years or older
Weight :	les than 5 kg	5-7,9 kg	8-10,9 kg	11-15,9 kg	16-29,9 kg	30 kg or more
In ml :	200-400	400-600	600-800	800-1200	1200-2200	2200-4000
In local measure						

* *Use the patient's age only when you do not know the weight. The approximate amount of ORS required (in ml) can also be calculated by multiplying the patient's weight (in grams) times 0.075.*

- If the child wants more ORS than shown, give more.
- Encourage the mother to continue breast-feeding.
- For infants under 6 months who are not breast-fed, also give 100-200 ml clean water during this period.

OBSERVE THE CHILD CAREFULLY AND HELP THE MOTHER GIVE ORS SOLUTION :

- Show her how much solution to give her child.
- Show her how to give it – a teaspoonful every 1-2 minutes for a child under 2 years, frequent sips from a cup for an older child.
- Check from time to time to see if there are problems.
- If the child vomits, wait 10 minutes and then continue giving ORS, but more slowly, for example, a spoonful every 2-3 minutes.
- If the child's eyelids become puffy, stop ORS and give plain water or breast milk. Give ORS according to Plan A when the puffiness is gone.

AFTER 4 HOURS, REASSESS THE CHILD USING THE ASSESSMENT CHART. THEN SELECT PLAN A, B OR C TO CONTINUE TREATMENT.

- If there are **no signs of dehydration**, shift to Plan A. When dehydration has been corrected, the child usually passes urine and may also be tired and fall asleep.

- If signs indicating **some dehydration** are still present, repeat Plan B, but start to offer food, milk and juice as described in Plan A.

- If signs indicating **severe dehydration** have appeared, shift to Plan C.

IF THE MOTHER MUST LEAVE BEFORE COMPLETING TREATMENT PLAN B :

- Show her how much ORS to give to finish the 4-hour treatment at home.

- Give her enough ORS packets to complete rehydration, and for 2 more days as shown in Plan A.

- Show her how to prepare ORS solution.

- Explain to her the three rules in Plan A for treating her child at home :
  - to give ORS or other fluids until diarrhoea stops ;
  - to feed the child ;
  - to bring the child back to the health worker, if necessary.

Treatment plan C to treat severe dehydration quickly

Follow the arrows. If the answer is "yes", go across. If "no", go down.

START HERE

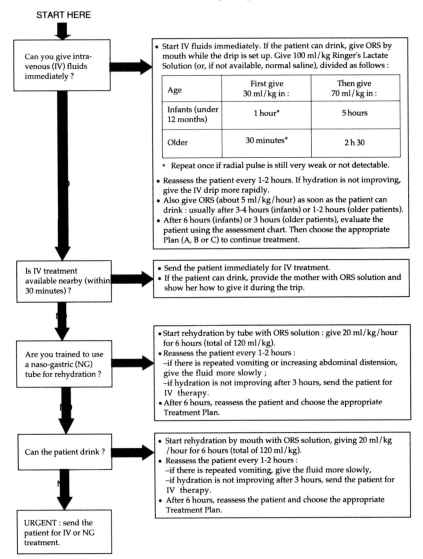

Can you give intravenous (IV) fluids immediately?

- Start IV fluids immediately. If the patient can drink, give ORS by mouth while the drip is set up. Give 100 ml/kg Ringer's Lactate Solution (or, if not available, normal saline), divided as follows :

Age	First give 30 ml/kg in :	Then give 70 ml/kg in :
Infants (under 12 months)	1 hour*	5 hours
Older	30 minutes*	2 h 30

* Repeat once if radial pulse is still very weak or not detectable.

- Reassess the patient every 1-2 hours. If hydration is not improving, give the IV drip more rapidly.
- Also give ORS (about 5 ml/kg/hour) as soon as the patient can drink : usually after 3-4 hours (infants) or 1-2 hours (older patients).
- After 6 hours (infants) or 3 hours (older patients), evaluate the patient using the assessment chart. Then choose the appropriate Plan (A, B or C) to continue treatment.

Is IV treatment available nearby (within 30 minutes)?

- Send the patient immediately for IV treatment.
- If the patient can drink, provide the mother with ORS solution and show her how to give it during the trip.

Are you trained to use a naso-gastric (NG) tube for rehydration?

- Start rehydration by tube with ORS solution : give 20 ml/kg/hour for 6 hours (total of 120 ml/kg).
- Reassess the patient every 1-2 hours :
  –if there is repeated vomiting or increasing abdominal distension, give the fluid more slowly ;
  –if hydration is not improving after 3 hours, send the patient for IV therapy.
- After 6 hours, reassess the patient and choose the appropriate Treatment Plan.

Can the patient drink?

- Start rehydration by mouth with ORS solution, giving 20 ml/kg/hour for 6 hours (total of 120 ml/kg).
- Reassess the patient every 1-2 hours :
  –if there is repeated vomiting, give the fluid more slowly,
  –if hydration is not improving after 3 hours, send the patient for IV therapy.
- After 6 hours, reassess the patient and choose the appropriate Treatment Plan.

URGENT : send the patient for IV or NG treatment.

Notes :
- If possible, observe the patient at least 6 hours after rehydration to be sure the mother can maintain hydration giving ORS solution by mouth.
- If the patient is above 2 years and there is cholera in your area, give an appropriate oral antibiotic after the patient is alert.

Management of the child with cough or difficult breathing

- **Assess the child**

  <u>Ask</u> :
  – How old is the child ?
  – Is the child coughing ? For how long ?
  – Is the child able to drink ? (for children age 2 months up to 5 years)
  – Has the child stopped feeding well ? (for children less than 2 months)
  – Has the child had fever ? For how long ?
  – Has the child had convulsions ?

  <u>Look and listen</u> (the child must be calm) :
  – Count the breaths in one minute.
  – Look for chest indrawing.
  – Look and listen for stridor.
  – Look and listen for wheeze. Is it recurrent ?
  – See if the child is abnormally sleepy, or difficult to wake.
  – Feel for fever, or low body temperature (or measure temperature).
  – Look for severe undernutrition.

- **Decide how to treat the child**

  – The child aged less than two months   see Annex 3a (page 31)

  – The child aged two months up to five years
    – who is not wheezing   see Annex 3b (page 32)
    – who is wheezing   refer

  – Treatment instructions   see Annex 3c (page 33)
    – Give an antibiotic
    – Advise mother to give home care
    – Treatment of fever

The child aged less than two months

SIGNS	• Not able to drink • Convulsions • Abnormally sleepy or difficult to wake • Stridor in calm child • Wheezing or • Fever or low body temperature	• Fast breathing (60 per minute or MORE) or • Severe chest indrawing	• No fast breathing (LESS than 60 per minute) and • No severe chest indrawing
CLASSIFY AS	**VERY SEVERE DISEASE**	**SEVERE PNEUMONIA**	**NO PNEUMONIA : COUGH OR COLD**
TREATMENT	• Refer URGENTLY to hospital • Give first dose of an antibiotic. • Keep young infant warm (If referral is not feasible, treat with an antibiotic and follow closely.)	• Refer URGENTLY to hospital • Give first dose of an antibiotic • Keep young infant warm (If referral is not feasible, treat with an antibiotic and follow closely.)	• Advise mother to give following home care : – keep young infant warm, – breastfeed frequently, – clear nose if it interferes with feeding. • Advise mother to return quickly if : – illness worsens, – breathing is difficult, – feeding becomes a problem.

Annex 3b

The child aged two months to five years

SIGNS	• Not able to drink • Convulsions • Abnormally sleepy or difficult to wake • Stridor in calm child or • Severe under-nutrition	• Chest indrawing	• No chest indrawing and • Fast breathing (50 per minute or MORE if child 2-12 months of age or 40 per minute or MORE if child 1-5 years)	• No chest indrawing and • No fast breathing (LESS than 50 per minute if child 2-12 months of age or 40 per minute if child 1-5 years)
CLASSIFY AS	**VERY SEVERE DISEASE**	**SEVERE PNEUMONIA**	**PNEUMONIA**	**NO PNEUMONIA COUGH OR COLD**
TREATMENT	• Refer URGENTLY to hospital. • Give first dose of an antibiotic. • Treat fever if present. • If cerebral malaria is possible, give an antimalarial drug.	• Refer URGENTLY to hospital. • Give first dose of an antibiotic. • Treat fever if present. (If referral is not possible, treat with an antibiotic and follow closely.)	• Advise mother to give home care. • Give antibiotic. • Treat fever if present. • Advise mother to return with the child in 2 days for reassessment, or earlier if the child is getting worse.	• If coughing more than 30 days, refer for assessment. • Assess and treat ear problem or sore throat, if present. • Assess and treat other problems. • Advise mother to give home care. • Treat fever if present.

Reassess in 2 days a child who is taking an antibiotic for pneumonia :

	WORSE	THE SAME	IMPROVING
SIGNS	• Not able to drink • Has chest indrawing • Has other danger signs		• Less fever • Eating better • Breathing slower
TREATMENT	• Refer URGENTLY to hospital	• Change antibiotic or • Refer	• Finish 5 days of antibiotic

Treatment instructions

• Give an antibiotic

 – Give first dose of antibiotic in clinic.
 – Instruct mother on how to give the antibiotic for five days at home (or to return to clinic for daily procaine penicillin injection).

AGE or WEIGHT	COTRIMOXAZOLE Trimethoprim (TMP) + sulphamethoxazole (SMX)			AMOXYCILLIN[3]		AMPICILLIN		PROCAINE PENICILLIN
	2 times daily for 5 days			3 times daily for 5 days		4 times daily for 5 days		1 time daily for 5 days
	Adult tablet single strength (80 mg TMP + 400 mg SMX)	Paediatric tablet (20 mg TMP + 100 mg SMX)	Syrup (40 mg TMP + 200 mg SMX)	Tablet 250 mg	Syrup 125 mg in 5 ml	Tablet 250 mg	Syrup 125 mg in 5 ml	Intramuscular injection
Less than 2 months[1] (< 5 kg)	1/4[2]	1[2]	2.5 ml[2]	1/4[2]	2.5 ml	1/2	2.5 ml	200,000 units
2 to 12 months (6-9 kg)	1/2	2	5.0 ml	1/2	5.0 ml	1	5.0 ml	400,000 units
12 months to 5 years (10-19 kg)	1	3	7.5 ml	1	10.0 ml	1	5.0 ml	800,000 units

[1] Give oral antibiotic for five days at home only if referral is not feasible.
[2] If the child is less than 1 month old, give 1/2 pediatric tablet or 1.25 ml syrup twice daily. Avoid cotrimoxazole in infants less than one month of age who are premature or jaundiced.
[3] Not included in kit but if available can be used as an alternative to ampicillin.

• Advise mother to give home care

 • **Feed the child.**
  – Feed the child during illness.
  – Increase feeding after illness.
  – Clear the nose if it interferes with feeding.
 • **Increase fluids.**
  – Offer the child extra to drink.
  – Increase breastfeeding.
 • **Soothe the throat and relieve the cough with a safe remedy.**
 • **More important : in the child classified as having "No pneumonia : cough or cold", watch for the following signs and return quickly if they occur :**
  – Breathing becomes difficult.
  – Breathing becomes fast.
  – Child is not able to drink.
  – Child becomes sicker.

> **This child may have pneumonia**

• *Treat fever*

• Fever is high (≥ 39°C)	• Fever is not high (38-39°C)	In a falciparum malarious area : • Any fever or • History of fever	• Fever for more than 5 days
• Give paracetamol	• Advise mother to give more fluids	• Give an antimalarial (or treat according to your malaria programme recommendations)	• Refer for assessment

PARACETAMOL doses :

AGE or WEIGHT	100 mg tablet	500 mg tablet
2 months up to 12 months (6-9 kg)	1	1/4
12 months up to 3 years (10-14 kg)	1	1/4
3 years up to 5 years (15-19 kg)	1 1/2	1/2

Fever alone is not a reason to give an antibiotic except in a young infant (age less than 2 months).

Give first dose of an antibiotic and refer urgently to hospital.

Sample monthly activity report

Diagnosis / Symptom groups		< 2 months	2 - 12 months	1 - 4 years	5 - 15 years	Adult	Total	%
ANEMIA	Severe							
	Moderate							
PAIN	Headache, joint pain							
	Stomach pain							
DIARRHOEA	More than 2 weeks							
	Bloody diarrhoea							
	Severe dehydration							
	Some dehydration							
	No dehydration							
FEVER	Malnourished patient							
	With chills							
	With cough							
	Unspecified							
RESPIRATORY	Severe pneumonia							
TRACT	Pneumonia							
INFECTION	Cold or cough							
	Prolonged cough							
	Acute ear pain							
	Ear discharge							
MEASLES								
RED EYES	(conjunctivitis)							
SKIN	Extensive wounds							
CONDITIONS	Limited superficial wounds							
	Severe burns							
	Mild, moderate burns							
	Severe bacterial infection							
	Mild bacterial infection							
	Fungal infection							
	Infected scabies							
	Non infected scabies							
URINARY TRACT INFECTION								
SEXUALLY TRANSMITTED DISEASE								
PREV. CARE IN	Anemia							
PREGNANCY	Malaria							
WORMS	Roundworm, pinworm							
	Hookworm							
Referred patients								
Repeated consultation for same diagnosis								
TOTAL								

Sample health card

HEALTH CARD CARTE DE SANTÉ		CARD No. CARTE No.	
		DATE OF REGISTRATION DATE D'ENREGISTREMENT	
SITE LIEU	SECTION/HOUSE No. SECTION/HABITATION No.	DATE OF ARRIVAL AT SITE DATE D'ARRIVÉE SUR LE LIEU	

FAMILY NAME NOM DE FAMILLE		GIVEN NAMES PRENOMS					
DATE OF BIRTH DATE DE NAISSANCE		OR OU	YEARS ANS	SEX SEXE	M/F	NAME COMMONLY KNOWN BY NOM D'USAGE HABITUEL	

CHILDREN / ENFANTS

MOTHER'S NAME NOM DE LA MÈRE					FATHER'S NAME NOM DU PÈRE	
HEIGHT TAILLE	CM	WEIGHT POIDS		KG	PERCENTAGE WEIGHT/HEIGHT POURCENTAGE POIDS/TAILLE	%

FEEDING PROGRAMME
PROGRAMME D'ALIMENTATION

IMMUNIZATION IMMUNISATION	MEASLES ROUGEOLE	DATE	1		2		BCG	DATE			OTHERS AUTRES	
	POLIO 0 POLIO 0	DATE			DPT POLIO DTC POLIO	DATE	1		2		3	

WOMEN / FEMMES

PREGNANT ENCEINTE	YES/NO OUI/NON	No. OF PREGNANCIES No. DE GROSSESSES		No. OF CHILDREN No. D'ENFANTS		LACTATING ALLAITANTE		YES/NO OUI/NON
TETANUS TETANOS		DATE	1	2	3	4	5	

FEEDING PROGRAMME
PROGRAMME D'ALIMENTATION

OBSERVATIONS / COMMENTS

GENERAL (Family circumstances, living conditions, etc...) GENERALES (Circonstances familiales, conditions de vie, etc...)	HEALTH (Brief history present condition) MEDICALES (Bref résumé de l'état actuel)

DATE	CONDITION (Signs / symptoms / diagnosis) ETAT (Signes / symptômes / diagnostic)	TREATMENT (Medication / dose time) TRAITEMENT (Médication / durée de la dose)	COURSES (Medication due / given) APPLICATION (Médication requise / effectuée)	OBSERVATIONS (Change in condition) / NAME OF HEALTH WORKER OBSERVATIONS (Changement d'état) / NOM DE L'AGENT DE SANTÉ

Guidelines for suppliers

Quality

1. The quality of the drugs must comply with internationally recognized pharmacopoeial standards.

2. At the time of shipment the product shall have at least two thirds of its shelf life.

3. Tablets should preferably be divisible and carry characteristic symbols for easy identification.

4. Drugs should be procured only from those manufacturers able to produce documents meeting the regulations of the WHO Certification Scheme on the Quality of Pharmaceutical Products Moving in International Commerce.

Labelling

1. Labelling should be in English and preferably one other official language of WHO.

2. All labels should display at least the following information :
   - International nonproprietary name (INN) of the active ingredient(s).
   - Dosage form.
   - Quantity of active ingredient(s) in the dosage form (e.g. tablet, ampoule) and the number of units per package.
   - Batch number.
   - Date of manufacture.
   - Expiry date (in clear language, not in code).
   - Pharmacopoeial standard (e.g. BP, USP...).
   - Instructions for storage.
   - Name and address of the manufacturer.

3. A printed label on each ampoule should contain the following :
   - INN of the active ingredient(s).
   - Quantity of the active ingredient.
   - Batch number.
   - Name of the manufacturer.
   - Expiry date.
   The full label should again appear on the collective package.

4. Directions for use, warnings and precautions may be given in leaflets (package inserts). However, such leaflets should be considered as a supplement to labelling and not as an alternative.

5. For articles requiring reconstitution prior to use (e.g. powders for injection) a suitable beyond-use time for the constituted product should be indicated.

Example of label :

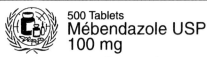

500 Tablets
Mébendazole USP
100 mg

Indication : Threadworm, Whipworm,
Large Roundworm, Common and
American Hookworm

Lot : 0158   Mfg : Oct 88   Exp : Oct 91

Dosage : Adults and children over 2 years : Threadworm – 1 tablet, Whipworm, Roundworm, Hookworm – 1 tablet morning and evening for 3 days. Should not be given to children under 2 years **Contra-indication** : Pregnancy.

Name and address of manufacturer

Packaging

1. Tablets and capsules should be packed in sealed waterproof containers with replaceable lid, protecting the contents against light and humidity.

2. Liquids should be packed in unbreakable leak-proof bottles or containers.

3. Containers for all pharmaceutical preparations must conform to the latest edition of internationally recognized pharmacopoeial standards.

4. Ampoules must either have break-off necks, or sufficient files must be provided.

5. Each Basic Unit should be packed in one carton. The Supplementary Unit must be packed in cartons of max. 50 kg. The cartons should preferably have two handles attached. Drugs, renewable supplies, infusions and equipment should all be packed in separate cartons, with corresponding labels.

6. Each carton must be marked with a green label (the international colour code for medical supplies in emergency situations). The word "BASIC" must be printed on each green label for the basic unit.

Packing list

Each consignment must be accompanied by a list of contents, stating the number of cartons and the type and quantity of drugs and other supplies in each carton.

The New Emergency Health Kit – WHO

Useful addresses

World Health Organization, Avenue Appia, CH-1211 Geneva-27, Switzerland. Telephone 41.22.7912111 ; telex 27821 ; telefax 41.22.7910746

United Nations High Commissioner for Refugees, Palais des Nations, CH-1211 Geneva-10, Switzerland. Telephone 41.22.7398111 ; telex 27492 ; telefax (general) 41.22.7319546 ; telefax (supplies) 7310776

UNICEF (UNIPAC), Arhusgade 129, Freeport, DK 2100, Copenhagen, Denmark. Telephone 45.31.262444 ; telex 19813 ; telefax 45.31.269421

OXFAM, 274 Branbury Road, Oxford OX2 7DZ, United Kingdom. Telephone 44.865.56777 ; telex 83610 ; telefax 44.865.57612

Médecins Sans Frontières, 8 Rue Saint-Sabin, 75011 Paris, France. Telephone 33.1.40212929 ; telex 214360 ; telefax 33.1.48066868

International Committee of the Red Cross, 17 Avenue de la Paix, CH-1202 Geneva, Switzerland. Telephone 41.22.7346001 ; telex 22269 ; telefax 41.22.7332057

League of Red Cross and Red Crescent Societies, P.O.Box 372, CH-1211 Geneva-19, Switzerland. Telephone 41.22.7345580 ; telex 22555 ; telefax 41.22.7330395

Christian Medical Commission of the World Council of Churches, P.O.Box 66, CH-1211 Geneva-20, Switzerland. Telephone 41.22.7916111 ; telex 23423 ; telefax 41.22.791.03.61

London School of Hygiene and Tropical Medicine, Keppel Street, London WC1E 7HT, United Kingdom. Telephone 44.1.6368636 ; telex 8953474 ; telefax 44.1.4365389

International Dispensary Association, P.O.Box 3098, 1003 AB Amsterdam, The Netherlands. Telephone 31.2903.3051 ; telex 13566 ; telefax 31.2903.1854

List of medications
(commercial and common names)

Acetylsalicylic acid = A.S.A., Aspirin

Adrenaline = Epinephrine = Levorenine

Aluminium Hydroxide

Aminophylline = Theophylline = Euphyllin®

Amoxycillin = Amoxil®, Clamoxyl®

Ampicillin = Amfipen®, Penbritin®

Ascorbic Acid = Vitamin C, Redoxon®

Benzathine Penicillin = Benzathine Benzyl penicillin = Penidural®

Benzonidazole = Benznidazole = Radanil®

Benzyl Benzoate = BBL®

Benzyl Penicillin = Penicillin G = Crystapen®

Calcium Gluconate

Chloramine = Tosylchloramide sodium = Clonazone®

Chloramphenicol = Chloromycetin®, Tifomycine®

Chlorhexidine + Cetrimide = HAC®, Savlon®

Chloroquine = Nivaquine®, Resochin®

Chlorpheniramine = Chlorphenamine = Teldvin®

Chlorpromazine = Largactil®

Cimetidine = Tagamet®

Clofazimine = Lamprene®

Cloxacillin = Orbenin®

Cotrimoxazole = Sulphamethoxazole + Trimethoprim = Bactrim®, Cotrim®, Septrim®

Dapsone = Avlosulfon®

Dexamethasone = Decadron®, Oradexon®

Diazepam = Tensium®, Valium®

Diethylcarbamazine = Banacide®, Notezine®

Digoxin = Lanoxin®

Doxycycline = Doxy 100®, Granudoxy®, Vibramycin®

Epinephrine = Adrenaline = Levorenine

Ergometrine (methyl) = Methergin®

Erythromycin = Erythrocin®, Ilotycin®

Ethambutol = Myambutol®

Etionamide = Iridocin®, Trecator®

Ferrous sulphate = Eryfer®, Ferro Grad®, Resofero®

Folic Acid = Folacin®, Foldine®

Furosemide = Frusemide = Frusid®, Lasix®

Gentamicin = Cidomycin®, Garamycin®, Gentallin®

Gentian Violet = G.V.

Griseofulvin = Fulcin®, Grisovin®

Hydralazine = Apresoline®

Hydrochlorothiazide = Dochlotride®, Esidrex®, HydroSaluric®

Hydrocortisone = Efcortesol®, Solu-cortef®

Hyoscine (N-Butyl) = Butylscopamine = Buscopan®

Indometacin = Artracin®, Indocid®

Isoniazid = INH = Rimifon®

Ivermectin = Mectizan®

Levamizole = Tramisol®

Lidocaine = Lignocaine = Xylocaine®, Xylocard®

Mebendazole = Vermox®

Mefloquine = Lariam®

Meglumine antimoniate = Methy glucamine = Glucantime®

Melarsoprol = Arsobal®

Methyldopa = Aldomet®, Medomet®

311

Metrifonate = Bilarcil®

Metronidazole = Flagyl®, Metrolyl®, Zadstat®

Miconazole = Dactarin®

Niclosamide = Tredemine®, Yomesan®

Nifurtimox = Lampit*

Nitrofurantoin = Furandantin®, Urantoin®

Noramidopyrine = Dypirone = Metamizol = Nolotil®, Novalgin®

Norethisterone = Norlutin®, Primolut®

Nystatin = Mycostatin®, Nystan®

Oral rehydration salt = ORS = Oralit®

Oxamniquine = Mansil®, Vansil®

Oxytocin = Pitocin®, Syntocinon®

Paracetamol = Doliprane®, Panadol®, Tylenol®

Penicillin G = Benzyl penicilline = Crystapen®

Penicillin V = Phenoxymethyl penicillin = Crystapen V®, Stabillin V-K®, V-Cil-K®

Pentamidine = Lomidine®

Pentazocine = Fortal®

Phenobarbital = Phenobarbitone = Gardenal®, Luminal®

Phenytoin = Di-Hydan®, Dilantin®, Epanutin®

Piperazine = Antepar®, Pripsen®

Potassium (Chloride or Gluconate) = Kalleorid®

Povidone iodine = Polyvidone iodine = Betadine®, Videne®

Praziquantel = Biltricide®

Prednisolone = Prednisone = Codesol®, Deltastab®, Prednesol®

Primaquine

Probenecid = Benemid®

Procain Penicillin = Procain Benzyl Penicilline

Promethazine = Phenergan®

Propranolol = Angilol®, Inderal®

Pyrantel pamoate = Combantrin®

Pyrazinamide = Zinamide®

Pyridoxine = Vitamin B6 = Becilan®

Pyrimethamine = Daraprim®, Malocide®

Quinine = Quinimax®, Quinoforme®

Retinol = Vitamin A = Ro-A-Vit®

Rifampicin = Rifadin®, Rimactane®

Ringer Lactate = Hartmann's solution

Salbutamol = Albuterol = Salbulin®, Salbutan®, Ventolin®

Sodium Stibogluconate = Pentostam®

Spectinomycin = Trobicin®

Spironalactone = Aldacton®, Osiren®

Streptomycin

Sulfacetamide

Sulphadoxine + Pyrimethamine = Fansidar®

Suramin sodium = Antrypol®, Moranyl®

Tetracycline = Abfosan®, Hexacycline®, Tetramig®

Thiabendazole = Mintezol®

Thiacetazone = TB1

Thiamine = Aneurin = Vitamin B1 = Benerva®, Bevitine®

Trimethoprime + Sulphamethoxazole = Cotrimoxazole = Bactrim®, Cotrim®, Septrim®

Vitamin A = Retinol = Ro-A-Vit®

Whitfield's ointment = 3 % Salycilic Acid + 6 % Benzoic Acid

Bibliography

1. AGREGES DU PHARO
   Techniques élémentaires pour médecins isolés
   DGDL Editions, 1983

2. ALLEGRA D. et Col. Emergency Refugee Health Care : A chronicle of experience in Khmer assistance operation 1979-1980
   Centers for Diseases Control, Atlanta, 1983

3. AMERICAN PUBLIC HEALTH ASSOCIATION
   Control of communicable diseases in man
   Abram S. Benenson Editeur, 1985

4. BERKOW R.
   The Merck manuel
   Merck Sharp and Dohme, 1987

5. BRIEND A.
   Prévention et traitement de la malnutrition
   Orstom Editions, 1985

6. BRITISH MEDICAL ASSOCIATION
   British National Formulary
   British Medical Association and the Pharmaceutical Society of Great Britain, 1987

7. CAMERON M., HOFVANDER Y.
   Manual on feeding infants and young children
   Orstom, 1983

8. DAWSON C.R., JONES B.R., TARIZZO M.L.
   Guide pour la lutte contre le trachome
   W.H.O., Geneva, 1981

9. FERRIER E.
   Précis de Pédiatrie
   Payot Edit., 1982

10. GENTILINI M., DUFLO B.
    Médecine Tropicale
    Flammarion Sciences, 1986

11. JELLIFE D.B., STANFIELD P.I.
    Diseases of Children in the Subtropics and Tropics
    Edward Arnold, 1978

12. H.C.R.
    Manuel des situations d'urgence
    H.C.R., Geneva, 1982

13. HAROLD FRIEDMAN H.
    Manuel de diagnostic médical
    Mesdi Editions, 1984

14. HERCBERG S. et Col.
    Nutrition et Santé Publique
    Lavoisier Paris, 1986

15. HUAULT G., LABRUNE B.
    Pédiatrie d'urgence
    Flammarion Médecine Sciences, 1981

16. KENNETH R., NISWANDER
    Manuel d'obstétrique
    Mesdi Edition, 1985

17. KERNBAUM S.
    Eléments de Pathologie Infectieuse
    Simep - Specia, 1982

18. KING M.
    Primary Child Care
    Oxford Medical Publications, 1983

19. Malawi Ministry of Health
    Guideline for management of malaria
    Ministry of Health, Malawi, 1986

20. MANSON BAHR
    Manson's tropical diseases
    Bailliere and Tindall Edition, 1982

21. MARTINDALE
    The extra pharmacopœia
    The Pharmaceutical press, London, 1982

22. MEDECINS SANS FRONTIERES
    Essential drugs – practical guidelines
    Editions Hatier, Paris, 1993

23. MEDECINS SANS FRONTIERES
    Principales conduites à tenir en dispensaire - Niveau auxiliaire médical
    Médecins sans Frontières, Paris, 1990

24. MORLEY D.
    Pédiatrie dans les pays en voie de développement
    Flammarion Médecine Sciences 1977

25. O.M.S./W.H.O.
    Fièvre hémorragique virale
    Technical report n°721, OMS, Geneva, 1985

26. O.M.S./W.H.O.
    La lutte contre la carence en Vitamine A et la Xérophtalmie
    Technical report n°672, OMS, Geneva, 1982

27. O.M.S./W.H.O.
La situation du paludisme dans le monde en 1990, parties I et II
Relevé épidémiologique hebdomadaire, 67 (22/23)
WHO, Geneva, 1992

28. O.M.S./W.H.O.
Voyages internationaux et santé – Vaccinations et conseils d'hygiène : situation
au 01/01/91
WHO, Geneva, 1991

29. O.M.S./W.H.O.
Manuel pour la lutte contre la trypanosomiase
WHO, Geneva, 1983

30. O.M.S./W.H.O.
Comité d'experts de la rage - Rapports techniques N°709
WHO, Geneva, 1984

31. O.M.S./W.H.O.
Nutrition in preventive medicine
WHO, Geneva, 1976

32. O.M.S./W.H.O.
L'utilisation des médicaments essentiels
Technical report n° 722 - WHO, Geneva, 1985

33. O.M.S./W.H.O.
La lutte contre les maladies sexuellement transmissibles
WHO, Geneva, 1986

34. O.M.S./W.H.O.
Prévention and Control of Yellow Fever in Africa
WHO, Geneva, 1986

35. O.M.S./W.H.O.
Traitement et prévention des diarrhées aiguës : directives destinées aux
instructeurs des agents de santé
WHO, Geneva, 1985

36. O.M.S./W.H.O.
Programme for the control of diarrhoeal disease – a manual for the treatment of
diarrhoea
WHO/CDD/SER/80.2 REV. 2, Geneva, 1990

37. O.M.S./W.H.O.
Programme de lutte contre les maladies diarrhéiques : directives pour une
enquête par sondage sur les taux de morbidité, de mortalité et de traitement
relatifs aux maladies diarrhéiques
OMS/LMD/SER/84.6 REVI, Geneva, 1984

38. O.M.S./W.H.O.
Respiratory infections in children : management at small hospitals
Background notes and a manual for doctors
WHO, Geneva, 1986

39. OXFAM
    Guide pratique de programmes sélectifs d'alimentation
    OXFAM, 1984

40. OXFAM
    Guidelines for tuberculosis control programmes in developing countries
    OXFAM, 1985

41. PECHERE J.C. et Col.
    Les infections
    EDISEM, Maloine, Paris, 1985

42. PENE P., ANDRE JL, ROUGEMONT A.
    Santé et Médecine en Afrique Tropicale
    Doin Edition, 1980

43. PERELMAN R.
    Pédiatrie pratique
    Maloine Editeur, 1977

44. PERINE P.L. et Col.
    Manuel des tréponématoses endémiques
    OMS, Genève, 1985

45. PERRIN Pierre
    Assistance médicale en situation d'urgence
    C.I.C.R., 1984

46. PETERSDORF, ADAMS, BRAUNWALD, ISSELBACHER, MARTIN, WILSON
    Harrison's principles of internal medicine
    Internal student association, 1983

47. REESE R.E. et DOUGLAS R.G.
    A practical approach to infectious diseases
    Little Brown and Company, Boston/Toronto, 1986

48. ROTSART, HERTHING I., COURTEJOIE J.
    Maternité et Santé
    Bureau d'Etudes et de Recherches pour la promotion de Santé Zaïre, 1983

49. SIMMONDS S. et Col.
    Refugee community health care
    Ross Oxford Medical publications, 1983

50. UNICEF
    Assisting in emergencies
    UNICEF, New York, 1986

51. WARREN K.S., MAHMOUD A.F.
    Tropical and geographical medicine
    Mc Graw Hill Book Company, New York, 1984

Index

FRANCE	Médecins Sans Frontières 8 rue Saint-Sabin – 75544 Paris Cedex 11 Tel. : (33) 1– 40.21.29.29 – Fax : (33) 1– 48.06.68.68 Telex (042) 214360 MSF F
BELGIUM	Médecins Sans Frontières 24 rue Deschampheleer – 1080 Bruxelles Tel. : (32) 2– 414.03.00 – Fax : (32) 2– 411.82.60 Telex : (046) 63607 MSF B
NETHERLANDS	Artsen Zonder Grenzen Postadres - Postbus 10014 – 1001 EA Amsterdam Tel. : (31) 20– 520.87.00 – Fax : (31) 20– 620.51.70 Telex : (044) 10773 MSF NL
SWITZERLAND	Médecins Sans Frontières 3 Clos de la Fonderie – 1227 Carouge / Genève Tel. : (41) 22– 300.44.45 – Fax : (41) 22– 300.44.14 Telex : (045) 421927 MSF CH
SPAIN	Médicos Sin Fronteras Avenida Portal del Angel, n°1, 1 – 08002 Barcelona Tel. : (34) 3– 412.52.52 – Fax : (34) 3– 302.28.89 Telex : (052) 97309 MSF E
LUXEMBOURG	Médecins Sans Frontières 70 route de Luxembourg – L-7240 Bereldange Tel. : (352) 33.25.15 – Fax : (352) 33.51.33 Telex : (0402) 60811 MSF LU
GREECE	Giatri Horis Synora 11 A. Paioniou – 10440 Athenes Tel. : (30) 1– 88.35.334 – Fax : (30) 1– 88.29.988

Imprimé en France par ISI, 75011 Paris
Dépôt légal n°9288 - janvier 1994